Criminology of Poisoning Contexts

Michael Farrell

Criminology of Poisoning Contexts

Warfare, Terrorism, Assassination and Other Homicides

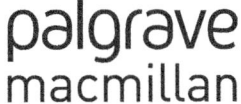

Michael Farrell
Stoke Lacy, Herefordshire, UK

ISBN 978-3-030-40829-9   ISBN 978-3-030-40830-5   (eBook)
https://doi.org/10.1007/978-3-030-40830-5

This Palgrave Macmillan imprint is published by the registered company Springer Nature Switzerland AG.
The registered company address is: Gewerbestrasse 11, 6330 Cham, Switzerland

Preface

I am delighted to be writing a preface to this third book on poisoning. *Criminology of Homicidal Poisoning* (Springer, 2017) examined many individual cases of homicidal poisoning and included some cases of serial poisoning. *Criminology of Serial Poisoners* (Palgrave, 2018) focused exclusively on serial poisoners. This book proposes a criminology of poisoning in different contexts: healthcare serial poisoning, assassination, terrorism, warfare, mass suicide, and capital punishment. Taken together the books constitute a comprehensive attempt to understand the role of poisons in homicides including theoretical frameworks.

I would be pleased to received comments that might strengthen future editions at my e-mail address drmjfarrell@bulldog1870.plus.com.

Herefordshire, UK							Michael Farrell
March 2020

Acknowledgements

It was a great pleasure to work again with editor Josie Taylor and the team at Palgrave Macmillan. Colleagues were generous with their support and advice. Regarding specific chapters, I would like to warmly thank the following.

Historian, broadcaster, and writer Mark Urban kindly commented on sources for the chapter on assassination. Prof Graeme Newman, University at Albany, the State University of New York, gave invaluable suggestions on a draft of the chapter on terrorism. Discussions with a former member of the Special Air Services, United Kingdom, were especially helpful with the chapter on warfare. Rick Ross, the Cult Education Institute, New Jersey, drew my attention to useful material in relation to chapter on mass suicides and cults. The staff of the British Library, London, were exemplary in their support.

Thank you again to all concerned. It should almost go without saying that any shortcomings of the book are my own responsibility.

Contents

About the Author

Michael Farrell was educated in the United Kingdom. After training as a teacher at Bishop Grosseteste College, Lincoln, and obtaining an honours degree from Nottingham University, he earned an MA degree in Education and Psychology from the Institute of Education, London University. Subsequently, he carried out research for an MPhil at the Institute of Psychiatry, London, and for a PhD under the auspices of the Medical Research Council Cognitive Development Unit and London University.

Professionally, Michael Farrell held senior posts in schools and units for people with various mental disorders. He managed a UK-wide psychometric project for City University, London, and directed a national initial teacher-training project for the UK Government Department of Education. For over a decade, he led teams inspecting mainstream and special schools and units (boarding, day, hospital, psychiatric). Currently, he works as a private consultant with a range of clients and has lectured or provided consultancy services in various countries including China, Japan, the Seychelles, Australia, Peru, Sweden, the Emirates, and the United Kingdom.

He has contributed to radio and television programmes in the United Kingdom and elsewhere and has written articles on crime and poisoning in a range of medical, psychological, police, and legal journals. His many books on mental disorders are translated into European and Asian languages.

1

Poisoning and Its Contexts

Introduction

We begin by defining criminology, homicide, and poison. With reference to different contexts (healthcare serial poisoning, assassination, terrorism, warfare, mass suicide, and capital punishment) I describe associated poisons. While emphasising the importance of theory and Situational Crime Prevention (SCP), I touch on the related criminological features of means, motive, opportunity, location, and perpetrator-victim relationships. The chapter next sets out the aims, scope, and features of the book. I describe its methodology and specify the proposed readers. Finally, to help give an orientation to the whole book, the subsequent chapters are outlined.

© The Author(s) 2020
M. Farrell, *Criminology of Poisoning Contexts*,
https://doi.org/10.1007/978-3-030-40830-5_1

Criminology, Homicide, and Poison

Criminology

In some perspectives, criminology is multidisciplinary, being informed by a range of social sciences. These include sociology, social theory, psychology, history, economics, and political science. As such a collection of disciplinary tributaries, criminology is concerned with the nature of crime, its antecedents, and the conditions that create crime as a social phenomenon (Lacey and Zedner 2012, p. 160). Others emphasise that criminology is shaped less by theoretical assumptions and more by its remit. In this view, it is the study of crime that makes criminology a coherent discipline bringing together practitioners including sociologists, social policy analysts, social anthropologists, psychologists, psychiatrists, statisticians, lawyers, and economists (Rock 2012, p. 70). In short, criminology is a multidisciplinary subject which may have different theoretical bases and is concerned with crime, its precursors, and its context.

Homicide

Law in England and Wales illustrates aspects of homicide common to many other countries. Homicide concerns the offences of murder and of manslaughter. It also applies to a person otherwise causing or being involved in another's death. Here the general criminal conduct or 'actus reus' is the same (killing another person) but complications arise about the causes (Croner 2008, p. 37). Under common law, murder is committed when 'a person unlawfully kills another human being under the Queen's Peace, with malice aforethought' (Ibid. p. 37). With 'malice aforethought' there is an intention to kill or to cause 'grievous bodily harm' 'Unlawful killing' includes, as well as *actively* causing another's death, *failing* to act after creating a dangerous situation (ibid., p. 38).

Certain special defences (diminished responsibility, provocation, and a suicide pact) allow for a conviction of manslaughter rather than murder, and a court judgement of 'voluntary manslaughter' (Croner 2008, p. 39). A court may make a judgement of 'involuntary manslaughter' where a defendant causes the death of another without the required 'mens rea' for murder, for example, by an unlawful act 'likely to cause bodily harm; or by gross negligence' (ibid., p. 41). The Corporate Manslaughter and Corporate Homicide Act 2007 provides that an organisation is guilty of an offence if the way that its activities are managed and organised 'causes a person's death' and 'amounts to a gross breach of a relevant duty of care owed by the organisation to the deceased' (ibid., Section 1).

Various types of homicide can be designated. They can relate to perpetrators ('male perpetrated homicide'), victims ('infanticide'), circumstances and location ('domestic homicide'), and mode of killing ('shooting' or 'stabbing'). As Brookman (2005) notes, homicide is diverse, and its forms differ considerably in their nature and underlying causes (ibid., p. 279). Hough and McCorkle (2017) provide examples of the range of homicides. Dobrin (2016) presents an overview of homicide data sources. Poison homicide, the topic of this book, specifies the mode of killing as well as examining other features such as perpetrator, victim, and location.

Poison

Although defining poisons looks at first as though it might be straightforward, the concept is slippery (Farrell 1990). It is a maxim of toxicology that 'the dose makes the poison' (Kolok 2016, pp. 1–9). Morphine for instance is beneficial in small doses to control pain but deadly in larger quantities. Nevertheless, even lethal doses of morphine are still tiny. So, we can still say that poisons generally have a harmful effect in small amounts.

The notion of a poison as a harmful substance has to be qualified. Boiling liquids are injurious but are not considered poisonous because their effect depends on temperature. Swallowing powdered glass will harm you but its 'mechanical' action excludes it from any poison list. Some substances such as pollen or nuts can harm people who are allergic to them, but are harmless to others, so the substances of themselves cannot be considered as poisons. We might think of poisons as being taken by mouth, but of course, they can be absorbed in other ways, such as by being injected into the bloodstream or under the skin.

All these points lead us towards a suitable definition. A poison must be able to kill or do serious harm to the functioning of bodily organs or tissues. A small dose is harmful. Its effect is not dependent on mechanical action or temperature, or on individual bodily peculiarities. Poisons may be administered in different ways. Such considerations are reflected in modern-day definitions. In *Dorland's Illustrated Medical Dictionary* (Anderson 2007) poison is stated to be 'any substance that, when relatively small amounts are ingested, inhaled, or absorbed, or applied to, injected into, or developed within the body, has chemical action that causes damage to structure, or disturbance of function, producing symptoms, illness, or death'.

Poisoning Contexts and Associated Poisons

Different contexts are a main concern of this book: healthcare serial poisoning, assassination, terrorism, warfare, mass suicide, and capital punishment. Each of these is defined and described in its relevant chapter. Immediately below I describe poisons associated with each context. This involves some repetition, but I hope it is forgivable because it enables the reader to get a quick overview of the poisons associated with each context under its own heading. The sections can therefore be used as a quick primer when reading the relevant later chapters.

Drugs Used as Poisons by Healthcare Serial Poisoners

Healthcare serial poisoners tend to kill patients with overdoses of drugs, or the 'wrong' drugs. Types of medication used improperly to poison patients can be classified according to their usual legitimate use. They are heart drugs (digitoxin and digoxin, lidocaine, potassium chloride, epinephrine, ajmaline, amiodarone, sotalol); muscle relaxant drugs (mivacurium chloride injection, pancuronium, vecuronium, succinylcholine chloride); analgesics (morphine, diamorphine, pethidine, acetaminophen); and diabetic drugs (insulin, glyburide). Healthcare serial poisoners have occasionally used other substances including sodium hypochlorite—bleach (Farrell 2018). Below, I describe poisons used by healthcare serial killers and which are discussed within fuller case studies in a later chapter. They are heart drugs, analgesic drugs, and 'other substances'.

Among heart drugs, the alkaloid *ajmaline* (Gilurytmal), first isolated from Indian snake root (*Rauwolfia serpentina*), is used to treat conditions involving irregular or abnormal heart rhythm. *Amiodarone* (Cordarex), which increases the time between heart chamber contractions, is used to treat conditions associated with irregular heartbeat including ventricular arrhythmias (which are associated with improper electrical activity in the ventricles of the heart). *Digitoxin and digoxin* are powerful extracts of digitalis which strengthen each heartbeat and lengthen 'rest' beats. *Lidocaine* (xylocaine) is used for heart conditions including ventricular tachycardia (typified by regular fast heartbeat) and is also used as a local anaesthetic 'numbing agent'. As an antiarrhythmic drug *sotalol* (Sotalex) is prescribed for serious abnormal heart rhythms. Medicinally, *potassium chloride* helps to treat and prevent low blood potassium which can occur owing to vomiting and diarrhoea (e.g. United States Pharmacopeial Convention 2019). Essentially, many heart drugs affect the strength and timing of heart rate to counter cardiac problems and if they are used improperly this very action can cause death.

Turning to analgesic drugs, *morphine* (an alkaloid derived from opium) induces euphoria in patients who are dying and eases anxiety in conditions such as shock or cardiac arrest. It dampens down aspects of the central nervous system, so inducing sleep and depressing respiration. *Diamorphine* is a morphine-based drug.

Regarding 'other substances', *sodium hypochlorite* (bleach) from a cleaning bucket was used to kill patients receiving dialysis treatment. It was introduced into their dialysis lines by Kimberly Clark Saenz who claimed that it was part of a disinfecting routine.

Poisons Used in Assassination

Poisons used in assassination include VX, Novichok, polonium-210, and ricin. Both VX and Novichok affect nerve transmission. VX is a lethal nerve agent, generally an amber-coloured translucent oily liquid, developed in the United Kingdom in the 1950s. Odourless and tasteless, VX can be dispersed as an aerosol or vapour into the air and can contaminate water, food, and agricultural products. Absorbed by inhalation, skin contact, or by being swallowed it can cause death in minutes. VX interferes with the action of the bodily enzyme acetylcholinesterase. (This enzyme breaks down acetylcholine—a neurotransmitter—at the gap between two nerve cells so that the next nerve impulse can be transmitted across the gap.) Severe skin contact causes sweating, twitching muscles, nausea, vomiting, and weakness. It can lead to unconsciousness, seizures, and flaccid paralysis. It causes fluid to accumulate in the air passages and digestive tract. Ultimately the poison causes breathing to cease, and death ensues (The National Institute for Occupational Safety and Health 2011).

Novichok refers to several nerve agents developed by the Soviet Union, and then Russia, from the 1970s to 1990s. Variants A230, A232, and A234 are used militarily. A230 was developed for cold climates. A232 (a VX replacement) made from precursor chemicals outside the Chemical Weapons Convention is as a powder absorbed through the skin or inhaled. A234 can be a solid, powder, or liquid. Novichok inhibits acetylcholinesterase, preventing normal breakdown of acetylcholine a neurotransmitter. This increases the presence of acetylcholine at neuromuscular junctions causing involuntary contraction of skeletal muscles. Symptoms can include headache, nausea and vomiting, confusion, blurred or painful vision, and faecal incontinence. Respiratory and cardiac arrest can ensue, leading to death from heart failure or suffocation (Ellison 2008, p. 4).

Polonium-210 can be explained in relation to uranium. Uranium atoms decay slowly into other atoms including polonium, a radioactive element. Among isotopes of the element is polonium-210. Polonium is highly toxic. Polonium-210 damages body cells and the hereditary material deoxyribonucleic acid (DNA). It reduces the number of white blood cells, increasing susceptibility to infection. A visible effect is hair loss. Damage to the gastro-intestinal tract leads to nausea and vomiting. Liver, kidneys, and spleen are harmed as well. Ultimately, as organs are increasingly damaged, and resistance is impaired, death ensues.

Ricin comes from the seeds of the castor oil plant, the castor bean, and is a by-product of castor oil production. An amount of ricin equal to two millionths of body weight can kill. As little as one hundredth of a milligram injected into the bloodstream can prove fatal. Poisoning by ricin leads to internal bleeding and kidney failure. Symptoms include fading vision, abdominal pain, a burning sensation in the mouth and throat, and nausea. Vomiting and bloody diarrhoea ensue. As blood becomes increasingly affected, the individual may experience convulsions before death occurs (Audi et al. 2005).

Poisons Used in Terrorist Plots and Attacks

Among poisons used in terrorist attacks have been cyanide, sarin, and ricin. Regarding cyanide, although the salts potassium cyanide and sodium cyanide are inert, water or gastric acid immediately hydrolyses them into hydrogen cyanide gas. So, swallowing cyanide salts generates gas inhaled into the lungs and absorbed by the gastro-intestinal tract. A minimum lethal dose is about 0.7–3.5 mg per kilo of body weight. Cyanide inhibits the bodily enzyme cytochrome oxidase preventing the body from using oxygen, even though there is enough of it present. Death may be from respiratory failure because oxygen deficit damages the nerve cells of the brain's respiratory centre, and because the heart's muscle walls are affected. Exposure to hydrogen cyanide gas can cause unconsciousness in ten seconds and death in a minute owing to cardiac arrhythmias and ventricular asystole, which affect control of heartbeat. Symptoms include giddiness and limb weakness. The lips and face turn blue. Heart action slows and becomes irregular and soon after convulsions may occur before breathing and heartbeat cease.

Sarin (GB) is one of a series of nerve agents known as the G series developed following the first nerve agent GA made in Germany in the 1930s. Nerve agents are manmade compounds, most belonging to the organophosphate group of chemicals and being liquids which disrupt the nervous system's normal functioning. Nerve agents can be directly produced using toxic chemicals or made from 'binary' chemicals which, when mixed, react to produce the nerve agent required. While binary chemicals are safer to manufacture and transport, the final nerve agent may be less pure and so less effective than one made directly (Shea 2013, pp. 2–3).

Ricin comes from the seeds of the castor oil plant and the castor bean. Two millionths of body weight of ricin or one hundredth of a milligram injected into the bloodstream can kill. Ricin causes internal bleeding and kidney failure. Symptoms include fading vision, abdominal pain, a burning sensation in the mouth and throat, and nausea, vomiting and bloody diarrhoea. As blood is increasingly affected, death ensues, sometimes preceded by convulsions (Audi et al. 2005).

Poisons Used in Warfare

Military planners may group chemical weapons as nerve agents (e.g. VX, sarin), blister agents (e.g. mustard gas), choking agents (e.g. chlorine, phosgene), and blood agents (e.g. hydrogen cyanide).

Nerve agents are manmade compounds disrupting the normal functioning of the nervous system. Most are organophosphates and are usually liquids. Germany made the first nerve agent GA in the 1930s, followed by others known as the G series including sarin (GB) and soman (GD). In the late 1940s England developed further nerve agents, the V series including VX (the hardest to manufacture and the most lethal). Nerve agents can be directly produced using toxic chemicals. Alternatively, 'binary' chemicals can be made that, when mixed, react to produce the nerve agent required. While binary chemicals are safer to manufacture and transport, the final nerve agent may be less pure and effective than ones made directly (Shea 2013, pp. 2–3).

Blister agents (vesicants) cause skin blistering and while not usually fatal impair combat effectiveness because troops are either unprepared or must wear preventive equipment. Mustard agents are common types of blister agents, having a mustard or garlic smell. They are oily liquids that readily turn into vapour. Blister agents have their effects if inhaled or if they have contact with the skin or eyes. Some can pass through normal clothing, even burning covered skin. These agents can have immediate or delayed effects. Among symptoms are that the skin reddens and becomes painful before swelling and forming blisters. Liquid blister agents severely damage the eyes. High concentrations of the vapour damage the eyes which become very painful. Inhaling the vapour can harm the lungs including causing direct blisters, and high concentrations can be fatal (Shea 2013, pp. 4–5).

Acting on the lungs, choking agents cause breathing difficulties and permanent lung damage. Examples are chlorine, ammonia, and phosgene (a colourless gas). Typically choking agents are gases with distinctive odours. Choking agents cause injury when inhaled. Low concentrations cause chest discomfort or difficulty breathing, and may irritate the nose and throat, and bring tears to the eyes. High concentrations can cause lung swelling, respiratory failure, and death. Symptoms of lung damage can occur up to two days after the individual has inhaled moderate concentrations of a choking agent (Shea 2013, pp. 5–6).

Blood agents affect cells to impair the body's ability to use oxygen. Examples are hydrogen cyanide (a highly volatile gas smelling of almonds) and cyanide salts (odourless solids). These poisons work when inhaled or ingested, especially affecting the central nervous system. Lower concentrations of blood agents cause headache, dizziness, and nausea for several hours before recovery. Higher concentrations or longer exposure can cause convulsions and coma. Individuals ingesting high concentrations fight for breath, experience convulsions, and suffer heart failure within a few minutes.

Poisons Used in Mass Suicide

Mass suicides have involved cyanide and overdoses of phenobarbital as poisons. Regarding cyanide, water or gastric juices hydrolyse potassium cyanide and sodium cyanide into hydrogen cyanide gas. So, swallowing cyanide salts generates gas inhaled into the lungs and absorbed by the digestive system. The minimum lethal dose is minute. Cyanide prevents the body from using its sources of oxygen. Death may be from respiratory failure because oxygen deficit affects the brain's respiratory centre, and because the heart's muscle walls are affected. Unconsciousness and death can occur very quickly owing to cardiac problems. Along with giddiness, limb weakness, and blueness of the lips and face, heart action slows and becomes irregular and convulsions may occur before breathing and heartbeat cease.

Phenobarbital is a barbiturate which depresses the central nervous system. It is used to treat people with epilepsy, insomnia, or anxiety and to induce sleep before a patient receives anaesthetic. Overdoses cause symptoms reflecting depression of the respiratory and central nervous systems. This may be an abnormal breathing pattern, low blood pressure, constriction of the eye pupils, slow or delayed reflexes, and increased resting heart rate. The individual may become unconscious and comatose, experience circulatory collapse, and cease breathing before death ensues.

Poisons Used in Capital Punishment

Poisons used in capital punishment include hydrogen cyanide gas in the gas chamber, and a combination of drugs for lethal injection (sodium thiopental, pancuronium bromide, and potassium chloride).

A prison gas chamber uses hydrogen cyanide gas produced when a pellet of sodium cyanide is dropped into a receptacle containing dilute sulphuric acid. When inhaled this gas inhibits a key bodily enzyme. An enzyme is an organic substance which can produce chemical changes in other substances without itself being changed. Cyanide inhibits the key enzyme cytochrome oxidase. This inhibition prevents the body from using oxygen, even when there is oxygen present. Symptoms of cyanide poisoning are giddiness, weak limbs, slowed breathing, and face and lips becoming blue. Heart action becomes slow and irregular. After about three minutes, convulsions may occur and the individual's breathing and heartbeat cease. Cause of death is effectively suffocation, as the lungs no longer absorb oxygen (Farrell 1994, p. 202).

Several drugs sometimes described as a 'cocktail' are used in execution by lethal injection, each having a different role and effect. Sodium thiopental (Pentothal) is a fast-acting barbiturate used in surgery as an anaesthetic. A lethal injection dose (up to 5000 mg) is many times higher than the medically used surgical dosage (up to 150 mg). Pancuronium bromide

(Pavulon), a muscle relaxant, is administered in a dose strong enough to paralyse the lungs and diaphragm. This synthetic drug has been compared with curare. Again, the lethal dose (up to 100 mg) is many times the medically used dose (40–100 mcg per kilogram of body weight). Pancuronium bromide takes effect in about one to three minutes. Potassium chloride is a heart-regulating electrolyte that is normally produced by the body. In a lethal overdose, it stops the heart (Farrell 1994, p. 203).

Theory and Prevention

The present book although self-contained forms the final part of a trilogy. Earlier books examined theoretical frameworks relating to homicidal poisoning including examples of serial poisoning (Farrell 2017) and of serial poisoning exclusively (Farrell 2018). In the current book the focus is contexts of poisoning such as warfare and mass suicide. I utilise the approach of Situational Crime Prevention which in turn draws on various theories of behaviour and cognition (see Clarke 2018 for a recent exposition). SCP also crucially indicates preventive strategies such as hardening the potential targets of crime. Relatedly, well-known criminological features of means, motive, opportunity, location, and perpetrator-victim relationship are also important.

Aims and Scope of the Book and Its Distinctive Features

This book:

- Discusses the theoretical background to poison homicide, leading to a consideration of Situational Crime Prevention.
- Examines poison use relating to the contexts of healthcare serial poisoning, assassination, terrorism, warfare, mass suicide, and capital punishment.

- Analyses each context in relation to SCP to examine potential prevention strategies and how they are circumvented.
- Interprets for each context means, motive, opportunity, location, and perpetrator-victim relationship.

I examine modern-day examples of poisoning contexts. Included in the wide international scope are examples from the Americas, Europe, Japan, and India. Many of these cases have been reported in newspapers, books, articles, television broadcasts and interviews, and internet sites.

I aim for direct, plain language, avoiding jargon. Where technical terms are used, they are explained. As well as a separate theory chapter, the book comprises chapters on different poisoning contexts incorporating Situational Crime Prevention and criminological features. Each chapter is structured to aid the assimilation of its content. This scaffolding includes an abstract and key words, an introduction, structured headings and subheadings, a conclusion, suggested activities to encourage reflection and discussion, texts for further reading, and references.

Methodology

Examples and cases cited in the volume are largely modern day. Referenced sources with internet links where appropriate include books, book chapters, journal articles, national and local press reports, and biographies. Further sources are television news reports, encyclopaedias, judicial reports, public enquiry documents, unpublished research theses, declassified documents (such as CIA manuals), and accounts of court proceedings. Referenced sources include ones in English and other languages. Sources have been used that are both reliable and available so that readers can access relevant documents through libraries, bookstores, and the internet. Additionally, in the work underpinning the book, I have sought the views of specialists as necessary particularly in the United Kingdom and the United States.

Proposed Readers

I hope that readers of the book will comprise both academics and professionals and include:

- students of criminology (including those in classes dealing with criminal psychology and homicide) and their teachers.
- criminal justice professionals: attorneys, homicide detectives, pathologists, toxicologists, and other forensic investigators and those who support them.
- Military, anti-terrorist, and intelligence personnel and those professionally supporting them.

In its wide scope, this volume has relevance to criminology, law and policing, toxicology and forensic science, criminal psychology, military studies, and anti-terrorism. It covers issues having international interest which I trust will attract readers in English-speaking parts of the world including the United States, the United Kingdom, India, various parts of Africa, Australia, and New Zealand.

Remaining Chapter Outlines

Chapter 2: Theory and Poisoning Contexts

This chapter discusses the nature of theory. It then outlines theories that aid understanding of homicidal poisoning in criminal cases and relate to moral reasoning, strain, control, labelling, differential reinforcement, and rational choice. I consider the relevance of each theory to poison contexts: healthcare serial poisoning, assassination, terrorism, warfare, mass suicide, and capital punishment. Then, the chapter examines how each theory might inform crime prevention leading to a discussion of theoretical underpinnings of Situational Crime Prevention (SCP). I discuss aspects of SCP and describe the preventive strategies emerging from it such as increasing the effort necessary for perpetrators to transgress.

Finally, I outline the criminological features of means, motive, opportunity, location, and perpetrator-victim relationships.

Chapter 3: Healthcare Serial Poisoning

This chapter defines healthcare serial poisoning and discusses its prevalence. A historical review is provided indicating the occupations of perpetrators and the range of jurisdictions involved. I discuss selected cases more fully: German nurse Niels Högel who killed many hospital patients; Kimberly Clark Saenz of Massachusetts who poisoned dialysis patients with bleach in their IV lines; US nurse Charles Cullen who confessed to killing more than 30 hospital patients over a period of 16 years; and Dr Harold Shipman, a UK physician who killed hundreds of his patients over decades. These are discussed in relation to attempts to identify 'red flags' of concern, Situational Crime Prevention (SCP), and the issues of means, motive, opportunity, location, and perpetrator-victim relationships.

Chapter 4: Assassination and Poisoning

In this chapter, I define assassination including by poison. Historical examples are touched on including plots to poison President Tito of Yugoslavia. More recently, assassinations and plots include the poisonings of Sergei and Yulia Skripal in Salisbury, England, using Novichok and implicating Russian agents. In February 2017 Kim Jong-nam, the half-brother of the North Korean leader Kim Jong-un, was killed at Kuala Lumpur airport by assailants using nerve agent. Russian spy Alexander Litvinenko was assassinated with polonium-210 administered in a drink of tea which caused acute radiation syndrome. Bulgarian dissident writer Georgi Markov was killed in 1978 with ricin poison by the Bulgarian Secret Service.

These are considered in the light of SCP and of means, motive, opportunity, location, and perpetrator-victim relationships.

Chapter 5: Terrorist Acts Using Poison

Historical plots involving poison are discussed in this chapter, specifically the group Nakam seeking to revenge the deaths of Holocaust victims following the Second World War. More recently, terrorist poison plots and attacks have occurred in various countries. In the United Kingdom, Husnain Rashid was convicted in 2018, and Kamel Bourgass in 2003. Sarin attacks were launched in the city of Matsumoto in 1994 and on the Tokyo subway in 1995. In Chicago in 1982, potassium cyanide was introduced into Tylenol capsules. These incidents are examined in relation to Situational Crime Prevention, and regarding means, motive, opportunity, location, and perpetrator-victim relationships.

Chapter 6: Poisoning in Warfare

Reviewing poisons used in chemical warfare, this chapter discusses their effects. Historically, chemical weapons were used in wartime and in military conflict in the First World War, the Italo-Ethiopian war of 1935–1936, and the Sino-Japanese war in 1943. More recently, chemical attacks have occurred in Syria and Iraq. In Syria, these concerned Khan Sheikhoun, in 2017; Khanal-Assal, Aleppo in 2013; and Ghouta, Damascus, also in 2013. In Northern Iraq, the Kurdish city of Halabja was attacked in 1988. These attacks are examined in relation to Situational Crime Prevention. Finally, the chapter looks at means, motive, opportunity, location, and perpetrator-victim relationships.

Chapter 7: Mass Suicide Using Poison

In this chapter, I review definitions of mass suicide including by poison. I look at historical examples of mass suicide by poisoning. Heaven's Gate, a US cult, saw death as a way of entering the next level of existence. In 1997, some 39 members killed themselves in Rancho Santa Fe, California, by taking poison along with vodka and placing plastic bags over their heads. In the mass suicide in Jonestown, Guyana, in 1978 Rev Jim Jones instructed his followers to drink poison as an act of revolutionary suicide leading to the death of over 900 people. These deaths are reviewed through Situational Crime Prevention and in relation to means, motive, opportunity, location, and perpetrator-victim relationships.

Chapter 8: Capital Punishment by Poisoning

This chapter gives a brief overview of capital punishment. Procedures involving poisons used in the gas chamber and in lethal injection are described. Focusing on the United States, the chapter considers the design of the gas chamber, its procedures, the prevalence of its use, and the course of an individual case that led to execution. Similarly, the chapter discusses the execution chamber for lethal injection, its protocols, prevalence, and individual cases of execution. I discuss SCP in relation to the death penalty by poisoning, focusing not on preventing crime perpetrated by the condemned person, but on structuring arguments against the death penalty and its prevention. Means, motive, opportunity, location, and perpetrator-victim relationships are examined in relation to the events leading up to execution by poisoning, emphasising the very particular circumstances.

Chapter 9: Implications of Poisoning Contexts

The final chapter summarises and reviews the various implications of using poison in different types of killing. I review the theoretical positions and implications for prevention. Means, motive, opportunity, and perpetrator-victim relationships are examined broadly across the different contexts. Implications of poison being chosen as the means of homicide are considered including how using poison shapes the activity and offers perceived advantages to the perpetrators. The chapter considers implications (relating to Situational Crime Prevention) of 'evasion' by the perpetrator and the 'response' by authorities and others.

References

Anderson, D. M. (2007). *Dorland's Illustrated Medical Dictionary* (31st ed.). Philadelphia, PA: Saunders/Elsevier.

Audi, J., Belson, M., Patel, M., et al. (2005). Ricin Poisoning: A Comprehensive Review. *Journal of the American Medical Association, 294*(18), 2342–2351. Retrieved from https://jamanetwork.com/journals/jama/fullarticle/201818.

Brookman, F. (2005). *Understanding Homicide*. London and Los Angeles: Sage.

Clarke, R. V. (2018). The Theory and Practice of Situational Crime Prevention. *Criminology and Criminal Justice*. Oxford Research Encyclopaedias On-line publication January 2018. Retrieved from https://oxfordre.com/criminology/view/10.1093/acrefore/9780190264079.001.0001/acrefore-9780190264079-e-327#acrefore-9780190264079-e-327-div2-3.

Croner, P. (2008). *Blackstone's Police Manual 2009: Volume 1 – Crime* (11th ed.). Oxford and New York: Oxford University Press.

Dobrin, A. (2016). *Homicide Data Sources: An Interdisciplinary Overview for Researchers (Springer Briefs in Criminology)*. New York: Springer.

Ellison, H. D. (2008). *Handbook of Chemical and Biological Warfare Agents* (2nd ed.). Boca Raton, FL: CRC Press/Taylor and Francis.

Farrell, M. (1990). What's Your Poison? *Solicitors Journal, 134*(29), 825.

Farrell, M. (1994). Execution by Poison Gas and Lethal Injection. *The Criminologist, 18*(4), 201–204.

Farrell, M. (2017). *Criminology of Homicidal Poisoning: Offenders, Victims and Detection*. New York: Springer.

Farrell, M. (2018). *Criminology of Serial Poisoners*. London: Palgrave Macmillan.

Hough, R. M., & McCorkle, K. D. (2017). *American Homicide*. Thousand Oaks, CA and London: Sage.

Kolok, A. S. (2016). *Modern Poisons: A Brief Introduction to Contemporary Toxicology*. Washington, DC: Island Press.

Lacey, N., & Zedner, L. (2012). Legal Constructions of Crime. In M. Maguire, R. Morgan, & R. Reiner (Eds.), *The Oxford Handbook of Criminology* (5th ed.). Oxford: Oxford University Press.

The National Institute for Occupational Safety and Health. (2011). VX-Nerve Agent. May 12. Retrieved from www.cdc.gov/niosh/ershdb/emergencyresponsecard_29750005.html.

Rock, P. (2012). Sociological Theories of Crime. In M. Maguire, R. Morgan, & R. Reiner (Eds.), *The Oxford Handbook of Criminology* (5th ed., pp. 39–80). Oxford: Oxford University Press.

Shea, D. A. (2013, September 13). *Chemical Weapons: A Summary Report of Characteristics and Effects*. Washington, DC, Congressional Research Service 7-5700. www.crs.gov RS42862 and https://fas.org/sgp/crs/nuke/R42862.pdf.

United States Pharmacopeial Convention. (2019). *United States Pharmacopeia [US Pharmacopeia National Formulary]*. Rockville, MD: United States Pharmacopeial Convention.

2

Theory and Poisoning Contexts

Introduction

Earlier work has examined theoretical frameworks relating to homicidal poisoning (Farrell 2017), including serial poisoning, in criminal cases (Farrell 2018). Such theories vary in their applicability to broader contexts of poisoning such as warfare and mass suicide. The widely used approach of Situational Crime Prevention (SCP) exemplifies various theories of human behaviour and thinking. From SCP emerge preventive strategies such as making it harder for perpetrators to carry out their crimes. Related to the theoretical background and the practical strategies are well-known features of means, motive, opportunity, location, and perpetrator-victim relationship.

The Nature of Theory

In general terms, theory is 'a formal statement' of the rules forming the basis of a subject of study, and ideas intended to 'explain a fact or event' (Cambridge University Press 2019). In science, a theory is a broad and

© The Author(s) 2020
M. Farrell, *Criminology of Poisoning Contexts*,
https://doi.org/10.1007/978-3-030-40830-5_2

systematic structure of concepts embracing empirical laws which concern 'regularities existing in objects and events' (Encyclopaedia Britannica 2019). A 'scientific theory' is a structure suggested by empirical laws which is developed to explain the laws 'in a scientifically rational manner' (ibid.).

A defining characteristic of science according to Popper ([1959]/2002) is its falsifiability. Accordingly, if observations are conversant with a proposed theory, it is confirmed. However, this does not imply that the theory will never be overturned. One incontrovertible fact disconfirming the theory requires it to be modified or replaced. A theory's adequacy depends on the correctness of the observations that it subsumes and predicts. Theory in the present volume resides between its common use and its more rigorous scientific meaning. It aims to provide broader explanations of phenomena than might be evident from initial observations.

Theory and Poisoning

Preamble

Among general theories of crime, several apply to criminal poisoning homicide including serial poisoning. These are moral reasoning theory, strain theory, control theory, labelling theory, differential reinforcement theory, and rational choice theory (Farrell 2017, pp. 29–42; 2018, pp. 30–38).

Moral Reasoning Theory

Moral reasoning theory (Kohlberg 1978) proposes that such reasoning develops sequentially and in parallel with cognitive and emotional maturity. It involves three levels, each with two stages. Level 1 is that of premorality. Its stages concern punishment and obedience, and a hedonistic preoccupation with one's own needs. Level 2 relates to conventional conformity. This comprises stages involving interpersonal concordance (associated with social approval), and a commitment to 'law and order' for its own sake. Level 3 concerns autonomous principles. Its two stages exemplify social contract and universal ethical precepts. As the person matures, the stages become more abstract. Offending is associated with the delayed development of moral reasoning, so that when individuals are presented with the opportunity to transgress, they lack the capacity to resist (ibid.). Accordingly, moral reasoning has been associated with criminal conduct (Palmer 2003).

In its application to different contexts, moral reasoning theory (Kohlberg 1978) could contribute to directly explaining healthcare serial poisoning. Concerning warfare, terrorism, and assassination, other factors including political ones might inform moral considerations. For example, wartime killing is seen in morally different ways by the victorious and the vanquished. Regarding mass suicides, moral deficits would likely be sought in those who encouraged and organised the deaths. With capital punishment, any assumed moral deficit might be placed not on the direct perpetrator (the executioner) but on the enabling legal system and the social norms supporting it.

In implicating offences with poor moral development, Kohlberg's theory implies that crime would be reduced if the moral development of individuals was enhanced. This points to possible educational interventions such as a programme of moral education in schools and other settings over a long period. Direct practical implications for specific crime reduction, however, are limited.

Strain Theory

Foreshadowing strain theory is 'anomie' (normlessness) (Durkheim [1893]/1964 and [1897]/1952). In one view of anomie, crime thrives when social disorganisation threatens societal collapse. Within this context, the social environment seems so disillusioning and debilitating that people could be led to 'commit suicide and homicide' (Lukes 1967, p. 139). In another view, crime develops owing to flawed social regulation which provides limited restraint or moral direction. For Merton (1938) crime emerges from tension between society's cultural goals and structural social limitations. In the United States, people were encouraged to pursue financial success, but individuals in lower social classes were often prevented from reaching such goals through the routes of education or employment. In response to the ensuing strain and frustration, in still seeking wealth, some people continue with legitimate aspirations despite not performing well. Others pursue deviant means like robbery (ibid.). These implications of anomie contributed to strain theory (Farrell 1991).

Adaptations of strain theory maintain that crime arises through tensions relating to unfulfilled goals not just of wealth but of achieving status and self-reliance too (Agnew 2001). This widens the theory's applicability to include homicide (Brookman 2005, pp. 103–104).

An extended strain theory (Agnew 2001) suggests a driving force for some acts of terrorism, some instances of healthcare serial poisoning, and even for an individual cult leader who guides disciples to mass suicide. Warfare, assassination, and capital punishment involving professional roles are less well explained. In strain theory, preventive implications suggest fundamental changes to social structure and markers of status. As such, they do not translate easily into practical approaches.

Control Theory

Control theory implies that many people would commit crimes in the absence of inducements to follow social rules, that is, if no effective controls existed. Hirschi (1969) suggested four inducements to rule compliance: attachment, commitment, involvement, and belief. To take just one example, attachment concerns to what extent some individuals respond to the opinions of others. Laub and Sampson (2003) studied the life course of a sample of men and how they resisted or accepted delinquency. The researchers examined how social bonds (e.g. friends, family, military service, and employment) form informal controls, filtering influences existing in the wider social structure.

A feature of control theory is the view that crime would increase if people lacked inducements such as attachment, commitment, involvement, and beliefs to comply with rules (Hirschi 1969). Yet, political and social forces can lead to people having ideas of attachment and commitment to their own territory that enable them to make war. Mass suicides may be incited where groups are isolated from normal social inducements. In capital punishment by poisoning the executioner is cushioned from any social inducements to desist, by legal structures and by the assent of decision makers. Other instances where individuals are little influenced by normal inducements may include terrorism, assassination, and healthcare serial poisoning

Importantly, control theory examines why most people do not follow a life of crime focusing on moral, social, and psychological aspects of rule compliance. Regarding crime prevention, control theory implies that society ensures that inducements to follow social rules are effective for individuals over time. Like moral reasoning theory (Kohlberg 1978), this suggests broad re-education, but does not point to practicalities of preventing specific offences.

Labelling Theory

Labelling theory draws on phenomenology and symbolic interactionism. In his transcendental phenomenology Husserl ([1913]/1982; [1913]/1989; [1913]/1980) maintains that we might doubt the independent existence of things, but not how they appear to us immediately in consciousness. Knowledge should therefore be based on these phenomenal experiences (see also Farrell 2012, pp. 49–53). Symbolic interactionism (West and Turner 2017) sees symbols as social objects derived from culture. People live in a symbolic environment. Indeed, the meaning of symbols is shared and developed in interaction with others. Through language, symbols become the means of constructing reality, mainly as a social product. A sense of self, society, and culture emerges from symbolic interactions, depending on such interactions for their existence. Even the physical environment is interpreted through symbolic systems in how it is made relevant to human behaviour (see also Farrell 2012, pp. 145–148). Accordingly, labelling theory seeks to explain how deviant acts and identities are constructed, interpreted, evaluated, and controlled over time. An individual commits an initial delinquent act ('primary deviance'), experiences the reactions of others identifying them as deviant, and responds confrontationally or defensively in a deviant role. In such circumstances, the deviance becomes 'secondary', incorporating the knowledge, stereotypes, and experience of others in shaping a person's identity and future behaviour (Becker 1963).

Labelling theory (Becker 1963) may partly explain aspects of terrorism, assassination, and healthcare serial poisoning. Here, perpetrators come to deeply identify themselves (especially with repeated offenses) with society's label. They see themselves as essentially a terrorist, an assassin, or a serial healthcare poisoner. If alienation from society contributes to people joining so-called doomsday sects, then self-labelling may reinforce feelings that suicide is a viable response to society's problems. Negative labelling of perpetrators does not seem to fit scenarios in warfare, where the opposing participants tend to justify their conduct. Neither does negative labelling fit the context of executioners carrying out capital punishment, as the prevailing legal system justifies their actions. Preventive implications of labelling theory include that the legal system (and wider society) avoids trapping offenders into a sole identity based on secondary deviance that gives little or no opportunity of 'going straight'.

Differential Reinforcement Theory

Differential *association* theory (Sutherland 1947) maintains that criminal behaviour is learnt in a social context. From this starting point, Jeffrey (1965) developed differential *reinforcement* theory. This utilised the notion of 'operant conditioning' concerning the effects of reward, punishment, and the avoidance of unpleasant circumstances on how frequently a behaviour occurred (Skinner 1938). In differential reinforcement theory, criminal conduct is 'operant' behaviour, determined by its consequences. A successful property crime rewarding the perpetrator 'positively reinforces' the criminal behaviour, increasing the likelihood of its being repeated. A poor person acquiring property through crime is enabled to escape poverty, exemplifying 'negative reinforcement', also increasing the likelihood of further criminal behaviour. Risks of being caught and the consequences of punishment tend to reduce the probability of the crime being repeated. As well as such physical or material consequences, social and personal repercussions act as encouragements or deterrents.

Hedonistic in implying that individuals normally seek pleasure and avoid pain, the theory has wide application. In some circumstances in warfare, killing the enemy is likely to reduce the chances of being killed or injured one's self. Given a certain set of beliefs and mind-set, a perpetrator can see an act of terrorism as rewarding in creating panic among participants in a hated political system. A professional assassin receives rewards of money or status for killing. Those who take part in mass suicides may see taking their own life as leading to great rewards in some supposed afterlife, or more prosaically as offering an escape from unbearable pain in their present existence. When a motive for healthcare serial poisoning is enjoying the power of life and death over a patient, homicide provides its own reward. Proponents of capital punishment, judges handing down the death sentence, and the executioner can all feel rewarded by the sense that they are supporting justice and retribution.

Preventive aspects of this theory are clear. If criminal acts are 'operant' behaviour they can be modified by altering the relevant encouragements and deterrents. Similarly, if a person's understanding of the risks and consequences of their actions is important, and these risks and consequence can be influenced, then that individual's actions are modifiable.

Rational Choice Theory

Sociologically, rational choice theory is about understanding opportunities for crime according to environmental variables. Psychologically, it views individuals as able to reason and to calculate risks. Rational choice theory proposes that people make reasoned decisions about committing crime, by evaluating opportunity and risk. Accordingly, the crime rate reflects factors influencing such decisions. Clarke (1992) delineates groups of circumstances that make it harder or riskier to commit the crime, or that reduce its rewards (ibid., p. 13, paraphrased). Factors making it harder to commit the offence include 'controlling facilitators' to reduce crime. Examples are restrictions on the sale of certain types of guns (or adaptations) to reduce gun crime.

Rational choice theory helps us to understand many contexts in which poison is used. In warfare, actions are determined rationally in the circumstances of specific military manoeuvres or strategies. Acts of terrorism, however abhorrent to victims, have a rational basis and planned goals for terrorists within their values and beliefs. Assassination too within a political sphere and guided by political aims claims a rational basis. Healthcare serial poisoning is sometimes seen by perpetrators as merciful killing. Capital punishment has a rational basis in ensuring that a perpetrator can never offend again and has justifications as retribution. Mass suicides, while incomprehensible to outsiders, seem to be a rational response for followers influenced by a charismatic leader or imbued with the teachings of a doomsday cult.

Preventive consequences are apparent in this theory. It identifies groups of factors (which can be introduced) that make it harder to commit an offence, that make it riskier to do so, or that reduce the rewards of crime (Clarke 1992, p. 13).

Theoretical Background to Situational Crime Prevention

As guides to preventing or constraining specific crimes, several of the theories considered so far are limited. Kohlberg's theory points to long-term re-education in moral reasoning. Similarly, control theory suggests broad re-education enrolling moral, social, and psychological aspects to ensure rule compliance. Strain theory implies making fundamental changes to social structure and markers of status. Labelling theory warns against the legal system and society at large, constraining offenders into a sole identity based on secondary deviance. In all these instances, the theories have good explanatory power, but are less adaptable to preventive action, tending towards long-term, broad, and diffuse approaches rather than strategies focused on specific crimes or problems.

Prevention is most strongly indicated by differential reinforcement theory and rational choice theory. As we turn to examine the theoretical background to SCP, we will see that rational choice and behavioural consequences make important contributions. In subsequent sections of this chapter concerning SCP, I am indebted to the description of SCP, its theoretical background, and its implications provided by Freilich and Newman (2019).

Deterrence Theory: Rational Choice, Agency, and Hedonism

Many SCP techniques are based on theories of deterrence, implying that the offender has certain tendencies and acts in specified ways. Individuals behave rationally and make rational choices. They have agency, that is, the ability to act independently. They also act hedonistically in tending to avoid pain and seek pleasure. All this is reflected in SCP strategies.

Some strategies endorse the effectiveness of warning individuals of the consequences if they offend, coupled with the relative certainty and speed of being apprehended. An example is the use of CCTV cameras (Cozens 2008). Other approaches recognise that legally shaped punishment is too deferred to influence most offenders' decision making related to criminal activity (Braga and Kennedy 2012). Punishment deters if it immediately follows the crime, suggesting that delayed consequences are ineffective. Accordingly, SCP endorses prompt or ever-present situational interventions rather than delayed formal punishment.

Some interventions make it harder for the crime to be committed, like fencing a vehicle parking lot so that offenders must scale the barrier to gain entry. This assumes that individuals will choose to conform because the increased 'costs' make it less worthwhile to offend.

SCP recognises that publicity can reduce crime. Publicising SCP interventions educate the public to take certain informed preventive or precautionary actions. These raise the 'costs' of a perpetrator offending by increasing the risk of apprehension (Bowers and Johnson 2005). Publicity can also influence offenders' perceptions of the difficulty and risks of committing a crime and the likelihood of being caught.

Behaviourist Interpretations

Some SCP strategies render it impossible for the offender to commit the crime despite their supposed motivation, mind-set, or emotions (Cornish and Clarke 2008, p. 41). For example, 'target hardening' through constructing physical barriers assumes nothing about the internal psychology of offenders. Nor does it require the presence of agency, rational choice, or a hedonistic nature. The individual is expected to respond to a given stimulus predictably, regardless of any supposed internal cognition and states (Newman and Freilich 2012, p. 216).

Triggering Internal Dispositions

Some 'soft' SCP approaches do not rely upon offender rationality or agency (involving conscious decision making) to reduce crime. Instead, they theorise that an offender has internal dispositions towards behaviours that can be provoked by certain characteristics of the environment. These dispositions may remain dormant unless certain conditions arise in the environment (the situation) that invokes the related behaviours.

For example, publicly displayed weapons (e.g. carried by a police officer) can cause some individuals to become violent, seemingly by provoking their internal dispositions. Without such stimuli, the person would not be disposed to offend. Related techniques aim to remove environmental cues that induce a person to offend. Consequently, in certain circumstances, this suggests police officers concealing weapons (Wortley 2008).

SCP, Social Class, and Culture

SCP takes a critical view of the concept of social class. SCP focuses on very specific and concrete (but not purely physical) situations. It therefore avoids social class interpretations of crime, regarding class as too abstract and as offering only vague preventive implications.

Differences in approaches are shown by studies of neglected, often city, neighbourhoods which tolerate vandalism and other minor crimes. Here, perceiving social control as weak, offenders may believe they can get away with more serious crimes (Wilson and Kelling 1982). This observation has suggested many preventive crime strategies for such neighbourhoods (Garland 2000). By contrast, a traditional sociological view of run-down neighbourhoods as reflecting lower social class would be too vague and would suggest impracticable policies such as re-shaping society (Freilich and Newman 2016).

A similar issue arises with the relationship between SCP 'situations' and culture (and subculture). In some types of organised crime, criminals embody values and behaviour codes, bringing to the situation convictions which form part of the circumstances to be assessed. But SCP in seeking to apply preventive techniques to specified circumstances can largely ignore whether a value is culturally based, providing that it is empirically identifiable and can be manipulated to modify decision making in a specific situation.

Freilich and Chermak (2009), focusing on extremist ideology, use responses shaped by the specified circumstances to prevent offending. This situational view of culture and ideology recognises that a situation imbued with profound cultural values can be modified. Known techniques are used that intervene in an individual's decision making at the right time, drawing on notions of guilt and shame (Wortley 1996).

Situational Crime Prevention: Its Development and Features

The Development of SCP

SCP aims to reduce opportunities for offending. It begins with analysing the circumstances which bring about very specific kinds of crime. The approach then uses 'managerial and environmental modifications' to change the 'opportunity structure' for those crimes to take place (Clarke 2018, abstract).

As a situational approach, SCP scrutinises specific types of crimes to identify aspects of the situation in which the behaviour occurs that encourages or aids the transgression. If the situation is at least partly a driver of the crime, it is inferred that altering or removing the situational encouragements will reduce opportunities for the crime to be committed. A perpetrator's motivation is not necessarily ignored. However, SCP takes the view that motivation to carry out a specific type of crime is influenced by the situation and the cues associated with it. Intention therefore declines where cues are removed, and preventive measures are seen as severely constraining.

SCP originated in the work of Ron Clarke. As research officer at the Kingswood Training School, a boarding school for delinquent boys in England, he analysed reasons why some boys absconded (ran away) from the school. Records revealed that aspects of the specific absconding situations provided opportunities for the boys to absent themselves. This 'opportunity structure' included seasons of the year when nights were longer, increasing opportunities to get away unseen (Clarke 1967).

If situations offered opportunity structure, one might develop interventions that reduce such opportunities and consequently constrain chances to offend, making room for Situational Crime Prevention (Clarke 1980). As researchers with police and others have focused on specific problems and situations, a raft of problem-oriented police strategies has developed (Arizona State University Center for Problem Oriented Policing, various dates).

Using a 'script' approach, SCP analyses the decisions and actions that an offender follows in carrying out the crime; a so-called 'procedural analysis' (Cornish 1994). Crime scripts involve chains of decisions and actions associated with reaching subgoals that contribute towards the overall goals of the crime (Cornish and Clarke 2002, p. 47).

Highly compatible with script approaches is a focus on the location of offences, supporting a geography of crime. Here, criminal events and behaviours are found to be patterned according to places such as street corners and neighbourhoods and associated with specific times (Brantingham and Brantingham 1981). Using such information, police or private security personnel may be able to intervene to prevent the offence.

Crime prevention can be built into the design of products and services (Ekblom 2012a, b). Product packaging and placement in stores may reduce theft, or even murder. The Chicago medication tampering of 1982, in which seven people died, led to all consumable products having tamper-proof and tamper-evident packaging (showing signs of interference).

Offender Choice

In examining an offender's choices (decisions) and actions, SCP assumes some predictability, implying that the offender's actions are not random and irrational. There is a context, however. An offender's perceptions of their needs and of environmental opportunities to conduct their course of action shape how they behave in a situation. Consider assassination. Here rational choice theory suggests that the perpetrator's perceptions of opportunities and constraints influence their actions. Likely, the means of assassination will have been highly rationally pre-planned such as deciding to use a gun to fire a poison pellet. But the assassin's perception will still rationally influence the action, for example the timing of the killing, and whether it follows the plan. In short, the assassin, and those involved in pre-planning, act to achieve their ends in what they see as a rational way, despite what an observer may make of events (Freilich and Newman 2019).

Specificity

SCP aims to prevent crime by removing opportunities for it, focusing on interventions to reduce specific offences (Clarke 2012). A crime-specific focus recognises that offenses vary in the context in which decisions are made. Situations in which crimes occur give concrete clues to the behaviour of the criminals, and indicate how this could be affected by changes in the social and physical environment. Focusing on a crime type or problem, analysts identify opportunities (situational characteristics) that allow the perpetrator to successfully complete the crime. Recognising such opportunities indicates intervention points where the offender's opportunities might be removed. When opportunities and intervention points are identified, preventive strategies are devised. In this way, prevention techniques are used to develop interventions to reduce crime in prescribed situations.

Opportunity Structure

Opportunity structure focuses on a specific crime and the application of the script method to find preventative interventions. Analysts examine the exact situations in which crimes occur, trying to identify the opportunities that situations provide for the offender to commit particular kinds of offence (Clarke 1997). Beginning with the situation(s) in which the crime occurs, analysts break down general settings into progressively smaller components. This may require collecting information from crime situation participants (e.g. offenders, victims, police). Such information addresses how the crime was committed, what helps it to be committed, and what barriers the offender avoids or overcomes. This enables analysts to map the opportunity structure of the crime and decide the point at which the offender's course of action can be deterred (Clarke 2012; Freilich and Newman 2016).

Techniques of Crime Prevention

The SCP framework comprises five general strategies, each embedding five crime-reducing techniques (Cornish and Clarke 2003). Hard and soft interventions are distinguished. Hard interventions can have two influences. They can deter offenders from committing the offense. Or they can make it impossible for the offender to commit the crime regardless of intent or level of motivation. Soft interventions reduce situational prompts that increase a person's motivation to commit a crime during specific types of events (Freilich and Chermak 2009).

The five general strategies in SCP are: increase the effort, increase the risks, reduce rewards, reduce provocations, and remove excuses. For each of these, five opportunity reducing techniques have been identified.

Techniques to **increase the effort** of perpetrators are 'target harden' (e.g. use tamper-proof packaging), 'control access to facilities' (e.g. baggage screening), 'screen exits' (e.g. documents allowing items to be exported), 'deflect offenders' (e.g. street closures), and 'control tools/ weapons' (e.g. smart guns).

Techniques to **increase the risks** are 'extend guardianship' (e.g. neighbourhood watch), 'assist natural surveillance' (e.g. support whistle blowers), 'reduce anonymity' (e.g. taxi driver identification), 'utilise place managers' (e.g. reward vigilance), and 'strengthen formal surveillance' (e.g. red light cameras).

Techniques that **reduce rewards** to the perpetrator are 'conceal targets' (e.g. unmarked bullion trucks), 'remove targets' (e.g. refuges for vulnerable people), 'identify property' (e.g. property marking), 'disrupt markets' (e.g. control classified advertisements), and 'deny benefits' (e.g. graffiti cleaning).

Techniques to **reduce provocations** comprise 'reduce frustrations and stress' (e.g. efficient service), 'avoid disputes' (e.g. separate enclosures in arenas for rival sports fans), 'reduce emotional arousal' (controls of violent depictions including pornography), 'neutralise peer pressure' (e.g. disperse trouble makers in schools and other institutions), and 'discourage imitation' (e.g. censor or restrict publication of details of modus operandi).

Techniques to **remove excuses** are 'set rules' (e.g. harassment codes), 'post instructions' (e.g. private property), 'alert conscience' (e.g. signatures for customs declarations), 'assist compliance' (e.g. litter bins), and 'control drugs and alcohol' (e.g. alcohol-free events).

When an analyst or a professional team are deciding on techniques to use in each situation, they review the empirical literature to identify previous relevant and successful interventions (Clarke and Eck 2005). From this, they shape new strategies (Ekblom 2012a). Which of these will be adopted and be effective depends on several factors like cost, how practical it is to implement them, and the extent of local community support (Felson and Clarke 1997).

Evaluating SCP Strategies

Two main methods are used to measure the effect of specified preventive interventions. The first, the script method, analyses the sequence of behaviours and events that are the result or cause of offender decision making. Opportunities and intervention points are highlighted, and interventions identified. The second methodology assesses the level of crime and/or change in the type of crime before and after the intervention. Some research uses time series analyses to investigate the impact of specific interventions, and has supported SCP's claims (Hsu and Apel 2015). Certain studies found a dramatic drop in crime after an effective intervention (Perry et al. 2016).

Problems of Displacement, and Benefits of Diffusion and Anticipation

One criticism of SCP intervention is that it will simply displace the problem and not reduce or eliminate it. Displacement can take place in different ways. The problem might cease to occur at a certain time, but merely be perpetrated at a different juncture. A different target might be selected for the crime. Although deterred from pursuing one type of crime, the offender may switch to another. Or the offender may change tactics to evade being caught. An intervention may lead to an offender moving criminal activity from one place to another (Reppetto 1976).

In some instances, there is a diffusion of benefits. An SCP intervention is implemented in one location, and the crime also falls in nearby areas or regarding similar targets where the intervention was not applied. Sometimes, anticipatory benefits occur, when a crime falls in an area while a proposed intervention is being discussed but *before* it is implemented. In both these instances, crime falls owing to publicity. Offenders hearing about the proposed intervention mistakenly believe that it is already in place in their area, and so decide to conform (e.g. Bowers and Johnson 2005).

Guerette and Bowers (2009) reviewed SCP projects, finding that 'displacement' and 'diffusion of benefits' occurred in a similar percentage of observations (26% and 27% respectively). Examining a smaller number of studies, in a similar way, the researchers found that when spatial displacement did occur, it was usually less than the treatment impact, so that the interventions usually reduced crime overall.

Further Criminological Features

Among frequently cited features when considering crime are means, motive, opportunity, location, and perpetrator-victim relationship. Each of these is important to individual criminal cases but are also relevant in wider contexts such as warfare and assassination. These features also relate to SCP.

Means

Among reasons for a perpetrator choosing poison over other forms of killing such as firearms is that the victim's death may be mistaken for natural causes, suicide, or accidental death. Other types of homicide are less likely to be mistaken in this way (Farrell 2017, pp. 131–133).

When we turn to contexts such as warfare or terrorism, similar questions arise as later chapters show. Here, SCP helps in analysing specific situations to see why poison was chosen and how this influences planning and perpetrating the homicide(s). In turn this can inform prevention.

Motive

Motives for poison homicide cases overlap with those for other homicides (Farrell 1990). A predominant driver is greed and monetary gain (Trestrail 2007). A further motive is to escape from a relationship, including a marital one, perhaps to shake off tyranny; or to gain sexual freedom (Farrell 2017, p. 139). Also featured are jealousy, and sadistic pleasure especially where the victim's death is particularly unpleasant and prolonged (ibid., pp. 139–140). A rare driver is factitious disorder imposed on another (American Psychiatric Association 2013, pp. 324–327). This is a form of abuse, usually of a child, in which a parent or carer causes or invents symptoms of illness in the child to attract admiration or sympathy for themselves (Farrell 2017, p. 140). In subsequent chapters, I will discuss motives for poisoning in various other contexts.

In some considerations of SCP, motivation is set to one side and the focus is on situational factors. Indeed, sometimes motivation is irrelevant where interventions make it impossible for an offense to be committed. In other interpretations however, motivation remains relevant. The motive to carry out a specific type of crime is believed to be influenced by the situation and the cues associated with it and therefore declines where cues are removed, and preventive measures are perceptibly highly constraining.

Opportunity

With criminal poison cases, opportunity has been limited by introducing legislation to restrict access to poisons including their sale and purchase. In England the vehicle was the Arsenic Act 1851 and subsequent legislation (Farrell 1989). Similar requirements were introduced in the United States (Trestrail 2007, p. 44). Criminals have evaded such restrictions, for example, by using easily available poison such as anti-freeze and by abusing professional (usually medical) access to drugs (ibid., pp. 42–44).

We will look in later chapters at opportunity in relation to many other contexts. Opportunity to commit a crime including homicide has a prominent place in SCP. It examines the aspects of a situation which increase or reduce opportunity to perpetrate an offence. Given that SCP sees situation as a driver of specific types of crime, altering or removing the situational encouragements is expected to reduce opportunities for the crime to be committed.

Location

Statistics on the physical location of poison homicides can be fragmentary. In the United States around 18,000 separate law enforcement agencies report certain aspects of homicide cases to the state level. Each state then aggregates the data to pass to the FBI who enter it in the annual Uniform Crime Statistics. State-level health agencies and bureaus of vital statistics report data on all kinds of recorded death cases. The Centers for Disease Control of the US government compile identified homicide deaths in a further aggregate report (Hough and McCorkle 2017).

Illustrative poison cases can shed some light on locations. A rural venue can involve poisons available in the locality including plant poisons, fertilisers, and pesticides. In an urban setting, poisons can be acquired from a factory or stolen from a large store. Reflecting the family origins of many homicidal poisonings, the killing may occur in the home. Further venues include places where medicines are stored and administered such as a nursing home, hospital, or doctor's surgery. Other places may be important, including where the poison was procured, prepared, administered, and discarded (Trestrail 2007, p. 70).

Location as later chapters show is a consideration in other poison contexts such as terrorist attacks and mass suicides. In relation to SCP and crime investigation, the location of a crime such as a homicide is often the starting point for evidence gathering and forensic work. Regarding crime prevention, different locations may be identified as being more likely venues of certain crimes—crime 'hot spots'. The broad notion of 'situation' in SCP includes crime location. Among strategies to reduce offending are analysing how the location might encourage it, then making changes to the location or aspects of it that are likely to reduce transgression.

Perpetrator-Victim Relationship

In individual and serial criminal poison cases, the relationship between perpetrator and victim is pertinent. Data from the 1980–1989 Uniform Crime Statistics suggested that many victims do not have a relationship with the offender, despite the expectation that most homicidal poisonings would take place in a domestic setting (Westveer et al. 1996). Illustrative poison cases indicate that perpetrator-victim relationships include those of actual and de facto family members, lovers and rivals in love, patient-medic, friends and former friends, and work colleagues as well as strangers (Farrell 2017, pp. 121–124). Perpetrator-victim demographics are important features of poison homicide and include gender, age, race, and social background/occupation (ibid., pp. 98–103 and 115–120).

As well as being important in criminal cases of poisoning, perpetrator-victim relationships and demographics can be relevant in other contexts such as warfare, terrorism, and assassination. For example, the relationship can be quite formalised as with that between an assassin and their target, and between healthcare serial poisoners and patients. In these circumstances, the relationship forms part of the SCP situation.

Conclusion

After reviewing theories concerning homicidal poisoning in criminal cases, a broad theoretical framework was suggested for contexts of poisoning such as warfare, terrorism, assassination, and others. Situational Crime Prevention (SCP) and related theories of human behaviour and thinking offer such a framework. SCP also points to practical steps towards prevention. Other criminological factors relate to the theory and practice associated with SCP namely, means, motive, opportunity, location, and perpetrator-victim relationships.

Suggested Activities

Consult the website of the Arizona State University Center for Problem Oriented Policing, https://popcenter.asu.edu/problems.

Look at examples from their list of *Problem-Specific Guides*.

Consider the typical patterns in approaches to problem-orientated policing, including closely defining and identifying the problem/crime, analysing the situational aspects of it, identifying approaches to reduce the incidences of the offences, and evaluating the results.

Key Text

Tilley, N., & Farrell, G. (Eds.). (2012). *The Reasoning Criminologist: Essays in Honour of Ronald V. Clarke*. New York: Routledge.

This book comprises various essays highlighting the contributions of SCP to policing, product design, and other matters.

References

Agnew, R. (2001). Strain Theory. In E. McLaughlin & J. Muncie (Eds.), *The Sage Dictionary of Criminology*. London: Sage.

American Psychiatric Association. (2013). *Diagnostic and Statistical Manual of Mental Disorders Fifth Edition (DSM5)*. Washington, DC: APA.

Arizona State University Center for Problem Oriented Policing. (various dates). *Problem Specific Guides*. Retrieved from https://popcenter.asu.edu/problems.

Becker, H. (2008 [1963]). *Outsiders: Studies in the Sociology of Deviance*. New York: Free Press.

Bowers, K., & Johnson, S. (2005). Using Publicity for Preventive Purposes. In N. Tilley (Ed.), *Handbook of Crime Prevention and Community Safety*. Portland, OR: Willan Publishing.

Braga, A., & Kennedy, D. (2012). Linking Situational Crime Prevention and Focused Deterrence Strategies. In N. Tilley & G. Farrell (Eds.), *The Reasoning Criminologist: Essays in Honor of Ronald V. Clarke*. New York: Routledge.

Brantingham, P. J., & Brantingham, P. L. (Eds.). (1981). *Environmental Criminology*. Beverly Hills, CA: Sage.

Brookman, F. (2005). *Understanding Homicide*. London and Los Angeles: Sage.

Cambridge University Press. (2019). Theory. *Cambridge Dictionary*. Retrieved from https://dictionary.cambridge.org/dictionary/english/theory.

Clarke, R. V. (1967). Seasonal and Other Environmental Aspects of Absconding by Approved School Boys. *British Journal of Criminology, 7*, 195–202.

Clarke, R. V. (1980). Situational Crime Prevention: Theory and Practice. *British Journal of Criminology, 20*(1), 136–147.

Clarke, R. V. (Ed.). (1992). *Situational Crime Prevention: Successful Case Studies*. New York: Harrow and Heston.

Clarke, R. V. (Ed.). (1997). *Situational Crime Prevention: Successful Case Studies* (2d ed.). Monsey, NY: Criminal Justice Press.

Clarke, R. V. (2012). Opportunity Makes the Thief. Really? And So What? *Crime Science, 1*, 3.

Clarke, R. V. (2018). The Theory and Practice of Situational Crime Prevention. *Criminology and Criminal Justice*. Oxford Research Encyclopaedias. On-line publication January 2018. Retrieved from https://oxfordre.com/criminology/view/10.1093/acrefore/9780190264079.001.0001/acrefore-9780190264079-e-327#acrefore-9780190264079-e-327-div2-3.

Clarke, R. V., & Eck, J. (2005). *Crime Analysis for Problem Solvers in 60 Small Steps*. Washington, DC: Office of Community Oriented Policing Services, United States Department of Justice.

Cornish, D. (1994). The Procedural Analysis of Offending and Its Relevance for Situational Prevention. *Crime Prevention Studies, 3*, 151–196.

Cornish, D., & Clarke, R. (2002). Analyzing Organized Crimes. In A. R. Piquero & S. G. Tibbetts (Eds.), *Rational Choice and Criminal Behavior: Recent Research and Future Challenges* (pp. 41–63). New York: Routledge.

Cornish, D. B., & Clarke, R. V. (2003). Opportunities, Precipitators, and Criminal Decisions: A Reply to Wortley's Critique of Situational Crime Prevention. *Crime Prevention Studies, 16*, 41–96.

Cornish, D. B., & Clarke, R. (2008). The Rational Choice Perspective. In R. Wortley & L. Mazerolle (Eds.), *Environmental Criminology and Crime Analysis* (pp. 21–47). Portland, OR: Willan Publishing.

Cozens, P. (2008). Crime Prevention Through Environmental Design. In R. Wortley & L. Mazerolle (Eds.), *Environmental Criminology and Crime Analysis* (pp. 153–177). Portland, OR: Willan Publishing.

Durkheim, E. (1964 [1893]). *The Division of Labour in Society*. New York: Free Press.

Durkheim, E. (1952 [1897]). *Suicide*. London and New York: Routledge and Keegan Paul.

Ekblom, P. (2012a). Happy Returns: Ideas Brought Back from Situational Crime Prevention's Exploration of Design Against Crime. In N. Tilley & G. Farrell (Eds.), *The Reasoning Criminologist: Essays in Honour of Ronald V. Clarke* (pp. 52–64). New York: Routledge.

Ekblom, P. (Ed.). (2012b). *Design Against Crime: Crime Proofing Everyday Products*. Crime Prevention Studies Vol. 27. Boulder, CO: Lynne Rienner Publishers.

Encyclopaedia Britannica. (2019). Scientific Theory. Retrieved from https://www.britannica.com/science/scientific-theory.

Farrell, M. (1989). Arsenic Poisoning: The Role of Legal Controls. *Solicitors Journal, 133*(35), 1101–1102.

Farrell, M. (1990). What's Your Poison? *Solicitors' Journal, 134*(29), 825.

Farrell, M. (1991). Strain Theory. *The Criminologist, 15*(2), 107–108.

Farrell, M. (2012). *New Perspectives in Special Education: Contemporary Philosophical Debates*. New York and London: Routledge.

Farrell, M. (2017). *Criminology of Homicidal Poisoning: Offenders, Victims and Detection*. New York: Springer.

Farrell, M. (2018). *Criminology of Serial Poisoners*. London: Palgrave Macmillan.

Felson, M., & Clarke, R. V. (1997). The Ethics of Situational Crime Prevention. In G. R. Newman, R. V. Clarke, & S. G. Shoham (Eds.), *Rational Choice and Situational Crime Prevention*. Aldershot: Ashgate.

Freilich, J. D., & Chermak, S. M. (2009). Preventing Deadly Encounters Between Law Enforcement and American Far-Rightists. *Crime Prevention Studies, 25*, 141–172.

Freilich, J. D., & Newman, G. R. (2016). Transforming Piecemeal Social Engineering into "Grand" Crime Prevention Policy: Toward a New Criminology of Social Control. *Journal of Criminal Law and Criminology, 105*(1), 209–238.

Freilich, J. D., & Newman, G. R. (2019). Situational Crime Prevention. *Oxford Research Encyclopaedias* (Criminology and Criminal Justice). Retrieved from http://oxfordre.com/criminology/view/10.1093/acrefore/9780190264079.001.0001/acrefore-9780190264079-e-3.

Garland, D. (2000). Ideas, Institutions and SCP. In A. von Hirsch et al. (Eds.), *Ethical and Social Perspectives on Situational Crime Prevention*. Oxford: Hart Publishing.

Guerette, R. T., & Bowers, K. J. (2009). Assessing the Extent of Crime Displacement and Diffusion of Benefits: A Review of Situational Crime Prevention Evaluations. *Criminology, 47*(4), 1331–1368.

Hirschi, T. (1969). *The Causes of Delinquency*. Berkley, CA: University of California Press.

Hough, R. M., & McCorkle, K. D. (2017). *American Homicide*. Thousand Oaks, CA and London: Sage.

Hsu, H. Y., & Apel, R. (2015). A Situational Model of Displacement and Diffusion Following the Introduction of Airport Metal Detectors. *Terrorism and Political Violence, 27*(1), 29–52.

Husserl, E. ([1913]/1980). *Ideas Pertaining to a Pure Phenomenology and to a Phenomenological Philosophy, Third Book: Phenomenology and the Foundations of Science* (translated from the German by R. Rojcewitz & A. Schuwer). Dordrecht: Kluwer.

Husserl, E. ([1913]/1982). *Ideas Pertaining to a Pure Phenomenology and to a Phenomenological Philosophy, First Book: General Introduction to a Pure Phenomenology* (translated from the German by R. Rojcewitz and A. Schuwer). Dordrecht: Kluwer.

Husserl, E. ([1913]/1989). *Ideas Pertaining to a Pure Phenomenology and to a Phenomenological Philosophy, Second Book: Studies in the Phenomenology of Constitution* (translated from the German by R. Rojcewitz & A. Schuwer). Dordrecht: Kluwer.

Jeffrey, C. R. (1965). Criminal Behaviour and Learning Theory. *Journal of Criminal Law, Criminology and Police Science, 56,* 294–300.

Kohlberg, L. (1978). Revisions in the Theory and Practice of Mental Development. In W. Damon (Ed.), *New Directions in Child Development: Moral Development.* San Francisco, CA: Jessey-Bass.

Laub, J., & Sampson, R. (2003). *Shared Beginnings Divergent Lives: Delinquent Boys to Age 70.* Cambridge, MA: Harvard University Press.

Lukes, S. (1967). Alienation and Anomie. In P. Laslett & W. Runciman (Eds.), *Philosophy, Politics and Society.* Oxford: Blackwell.

Merton, R. K. (1938). Social Structure and Anomie. *American Sociological Review, 3,* 672–682.

Newman, G. R., & Freilich, J. D. (2012). Extending the Reach of Situational Crime Prevention. In N. Tilley & G. Farrell (Eds.), *The Reasoning Criminologist: Essays in Honor of Ronald V. Clarke* (pp. 212–225). New York: Routledge.

Palmer, E. J. (2003). *Offending Behaviour: Moral Reasoning, Criminal Conduct and Rehabilitation of Offenders.* Cullompton, Devon: Willan Publishing.

Perry, S., Apel, R., Newman, G. R., & Clarke, R. V. (2016). The Situational Prevention of Terrorism: An Evaluation of the Israeli West Bank Barrier. *Journal of Quantitative Criminology, 33*(4), 727–751.

Popper, K. (2002 [1959]). *The Logic of Scientific Discovery* (Routledge Classics edition). Abingdon, Oxfordshire: Routledge.

Reppetto, T. A. (1976). Crime Prevention and the Displacement Phenomenon. *Crime and Delinquency, 22*(2), 166–177.

Skinner, B. F. (1938). *The Behaviour of Organisms: An Experimental Analysis.* New York: Appleton-Century-Crofts.

Sutherland, E. H. (1947). *Principles of Criminology* (2nd ed.). Philadelphia, PA: Lippincott.

Trestrail, J. H. (2007). *Criminal Poisoning: Investigational Guide for Law Enforcement, Toxicologists, Forensic Scientists and Attorneys* (2nd ed.). Totowa, NJ: Humana Press.

West, R. L., & Turner, L. H. (2017). *Introducing Communication Theory: Analysis and Application* (6th ed.). New York, NY: McGraw-Hill Education.

Westveer, A. E., Trestrail, J. H., & Pinizotto, J. (1996). Homicidal Poisonings in the United States – An Analysis of the Uniform Crime Reports from 1980 Through 1989. *American Journal of Forensic Medicine and Pathology, 17*(4), 282–288.

Wilson, J. Q., & Kelling, G. L. (1982). Broken Windows. *Atlantic Monthly,* *249*, 29–38.

Wortley, R. K. (1996). Guilt, Shame and Situational Crime Prevention. *Crime Prevention Studies, 5,* 115–132.

Wortley, R. K. (2008). Situational Precipitators of Crime. In R. Wortley & L. Mazerolle (Eds.), *Environmental Criminology and Crime Analysis* (pp. 48–69). Portland, OR: Willan Publishing.

3

Healthcare Serial Poisoning

Introduction

This chapter defines healthcare serial poisoning, discusses its prevalence, and considers historical examples. I look at the cases of Niels Högel, Kimberly Clark Saenz, Charles Cullen, and Dr Harold Shipman in relation to attempts to identify 'red flags', Situational Crime Prevention, and the issues of means, motive, opportunity, location, and perpetrator-victim relationships.

Definition and Scale of Healthcare Serial Poisoning

Ramsland (2007) defined a healthcare serial killer as 'any type of employee in the health care system who use their position to murder at least two patients in two separate incidents, with the psychological capacity for more killing' (ibid., pp. xi–xii). While this definition usefully specifies the perpetrator's setting and refers to at least two killings, reference to a 'psychological capacity for more killing' is problematic. Any such supposed

© The Author(s) 2020
M. Farrell, *Criminology of Poisoning Contexts*,
https://doi.org/10.1007/978-3-030-40830-5_3

capacity is difficult to demonstrate. Also important are healthcare settings and the roles of people working in them.

Settings can be hospitals as various as large multidepartment venues and small local 'cottage' hospitals, medical centres, clinics, community surgeries, nursing homes, long-term care facilities, assisted living provision, and patients' homes visited by medical and care staff.

Healthcare personnel are also varied. In discussing 'healthcare killers' as well as doctors and nurses, Hickey (2010) mentions 'orderlies, nursing assistants, and certified home health workers' (ibid., p. 168). Orderlies can assist patients eating and dressing, transport patients to different locations, and ensure that the venue is clean. Nursing assistants help clients under the supervision of a nurse. Home healthcare workers may assist with eating, bathing, lifting and moving, and self-care and may supervise clients in taking medication.

In the present chapter, I refer to perpetrators convicted of two or more poisonings of patients or clients, where there is an interval between killings (please see also Holmes and Holmes 2010, pp. 5–6; Hickey 2010, p. 27; Behavioural Analysis Unit 2005, pp. 8–9). This excludes healthcare professionals convicted of serial killing using methods other than poisoning, for example, suffocation. Also excluded are cases where healthcare workers have poisoned outside their role. I also leave out wartime state-endorsed killings including those of Nazi medics in Second World War.

Accurate estimates of the scale of healthcare poisoning are evasive. However, among single instances of poisoning, a disproportionate number of perpetrators have been healthcare professionals (Kinnell 2000). Furthermore, medicine is said to have 'thrown up more serial killers than all the other professions put together, with nursing a close second' (ibid.).

Historical Examples

Examples illustrate the international nature of healthcare serial poisoning and its persistence from earlier times (Farrell 2018). Nurse Jane Toppan of Massachusetts poisoned associates, relatives, and patients under her private care and was judged 'insane' (Reporter 1902). Medical porter Frederick Mors killed elderly patients in a New York nursing home with arsenic and chloroform and was also found insane (Ephemeral New York 2015). Coronary care nurse Robert Diaz injected patients with lethal doses of lidocaine at two Riverside hospitals. In Texas, Genene Jones, a paediatric nurse, injected children with succinylcholine and other drugs (Hickey 2010). Hospital worker Donald Harvey killed patients (including with cyanide) at hospitals in Kentucky and Ohio (Trestrail 2007, p. 23).

Nurse Bobby Sue Dudley-Terrell gave fatal insulin overdoses to patients at a Florida Healthcare Centre (United Press International 1986). In order to spuriously intervene and 'help' patients, New York nurse Richard Angelo injected drugs into patients' IV tubes to cause fatal respiratory problems (Associated Press 1990). Nurse Brian Rosenfeld killed three patients with Demerol overdoses (Reporter 1992). Dorothea Puente, a nurse's aide, then care home manager, poisoned patients with overdoses of drugs including Tylenol (Connell 2011). Physician Michael Swango killed at least four patients with arsenic and is strongly suspected of murdering others too (Stewart 1999).

US nurse Kristen Gilbert was found guilty of murdering patients with epinephrine injections (Farragher 2000). Respiratory therapist Efren Saldivar injected patients with lethal doses of drugs including Pancuronium, causing respiratory arrest or cardiac failure (Lieberman 2002). Nurse Vickie Dawn Jackson murdered ten patients with mivacurium chloride, becoming vengeful when other nurses showed them compassion (Associated Press, 3 October 2006). In Canada, nurse Elizabeth Wettlaufer murdered patients with insulin injections (McQuigge 2017).

UK nursing home manager Dorothea Waddingham murdered two patients (a mother and daughter) with overdoses of morphine tablets to gain inheritance money made over in exchange for their care (Glaister 1954). Nurse Benjamin Geen was convicted of murdering two patients at a UK hospital with drugs causing respiratory or hypoglycaemic arrest (Payne 2006). Colin Norris was convicted of murdering several hospital patients with insulin injections (Campbell 2011). Nurse Victorino Chua added insulin to saline bags so patients were unwittingly killed by other nurses (Scheerhout 2015).

Swiss nurse Marie Jeanneret administered belladonna (and other poisons) to kill patients likely from sadistic motives (Reporter 1884).

Exploiting victims fleeing occupied France, Dr Marcel Petiot killed them with cyanide injections, claiming they were vaccines required for their destination country (Maeder 1980). Christine Malèvre killed six patients at a Paris hospital with morphine and other drugs (Bryant 2003). Norwegian Arnfinn Nessett killed 21 of his nursing home residents with succinylcholine chloride (Wilson and Seaman 1983). German nurse Stephan Letter was found guilty of 16 counts of poisoning patients at a hospital in Bavaria, falsely claiming they were mercy killings (Cleaver 2006).

Situational Crime Prevention

Situational Crime Prevention (SCP) is fully described in Chap. 2. Five general strategies are each associated with five opportunity reducing techniques. Techniques to **increase the effort** of perpetrators are 'target harden', 'control access to facilities', 'screen exits', 'deflect offenders', and 'control tools/weapons'. **Increase the risks** concerns 'extend guardianship', 'assist natural surveillance', 'reduce anonymity', 'utilise place managers', and 'strengthen formal surveillance'. Techniques to **reduce rewards** to the perpetrator are 'conceal targets', 'remove targets', 'identify property', 'disrupt markets', and 'deny benefits'. Techniques to **reduce provocations** comprise 'reduce frustrations and stress', 'avoid disputes', 'reduce emotional arousal', 'neutralise peer pressure', and 'discourage imitation'. **Remove excuses** concerns 'set rules', 'post instructions', 'alert conscience', 'assist compliance', and 'control drugs and alcohol'.

Niels Högel, Germany

Niels Högel—The Case

Born in 1975, German nurse, Niels Högel worked in various clinics and a home for the elderly and was also employed by the emergency medical services. On 22 June 2005, he was working in a clinic in Delmenhorst, when a colleague reported to hospital authorities that Högel had given a patient an unauthorised injection of the heart drug ajmaline. Next day, the patient died. Before any preventive action was taken, another patient treated by Högel died on the evening of 24 June. It appears that hospital managers took two days before raising the initial concern with Högel and calling police. Högel's conduct began to come to light. Accused of attempted murder, he was tried, convicted, and given a seven-and-a-half-year jail sentence in 2008. As investigations continued Högel admitted administering unauthorised injections to around 90 patients, of which 60 were resuscitated and 30 died.

In February 2015, at a further trial, Högel was convicted of murdering two intensive care patients and attempting to murder three others. He was given a life jail sentence. Prosecution lawyers argued that Högel yearned to exhibit his resuscitation skills. Having injected a victim with a drug to induce heart failure, he would then step in to try to 'rescue' the patient with artificial respiration. Högel told the court that he became elated when his resuscitation attempts succeeded and downcast when they failed.

In October 2017, having exhumed the bodies of 99 patients, authorities judged 33 had died of a lethal injection. Police believe that Högel killed his first victims at the Oldenburg Clinic in February 2000 and went on to kill 35 more before leaving this post with 'glowing references' (DW News Report 2019). In 2002, Högel moved to Delmenhorst near Bremen, where he is suspected of killing 48 more patients (Eddy 2019). Oldenburg Police Chief Johann Kuehme criticised hospital delays in alerting the proper authorities (Oltermann 2017).

At a third trial from October 2018 to mid-2019 Högel was convicted of 85 murders and given a second life sentence in prison.

Högel used various medications, overdoses of which can cause potentially fatal cardiac arrhythmia and lowered blood pressure. These included ajmaline (Gilurytmal), sotalol (Sotalex), lidocaine/xylocaine, amiodarone (Cordarex), and potassium chloride.

Niels Högel—Analysis

Högel avoided strategies that might have **increased the effort** required to kill. Patients as *targets were not hardened* because possible warning signs were not recognised or acted upon. Any procedures to *control access to* *facilities* and *screen exits* had no effect because Högel had legitimate access to the hospital and patients. Similarly, *controlling tools/weapons* as applied to drugs was sidestepped because of Högel's access to medication.

Concerning **increasing the risks**, *formal surveillance* failed to detect potential warnings and lead to action. Any *natural surveillance* where staff expressed concerns was not sufficiently assisted. Indications were not acted on such as Högel's enthusiasm to demonstrate resuscitation skills, or the increased death rate at the Delmenhorst clinic. Even when Högel was seen illicitly injecting a patient, action was delayed and another killing took place in the interim. Oldenburg authorities appear to have missed the opportunity to *extend guardianship*. Indeed, Högel was given a clean reference when he moved to Delmenhorst Hospital despite some people in Oldenburg seemingly knowing of his abnormal behaviour. *Utilising place managers* includes enhancing supervision but seemed ineffectual perhaps because Högel knew from hospital routines when he could seize opportunities.

Turning to **reducing rewards** to the perpetrator by *identifying property* authorities did not identify and supervise the use of the drugs Högel used to kill sufficiently. This was because suspicion was not aroused early enough or was not promptly acted upon.

Regarding **reducing provocation** investigative authorities sought to *discourage imitation* once Högel was apprehended and details of his crimes gradually emerged. They aimed to alert hospitals and other facilities to the risks of such perpetrators, while not giving ideas to other would-be poisoners.

Removing excuses did not arise with Högel, who made no excuses for his killings but used them for self-aggrandisement.

Kimberly Clark Saenz, US

Kimberly Clark Saenz—The Case

Kimberly Clark Saenz (née Fowler) was born in 1973 at Fall River, Massachusetts, the United States. Married to Mark Saenz she had two children and was trained as a licenced practical/vocational nurse. She worked at Woodland Heights Hospital, Lufkin, Texas, but was dismissed for stealing the opioid pain killer pethidine/meperidine.

As strains grew in the marriage, Mark Saenz filed for divorce in 2007. From September that year, Kimberly was working at a dialysis clinic in Lufkin, run by Denver-based healthcare company DaVita. Concerns emerged. In April 2008, a letter from an anonymous official pointed to the high number of emergency calls for paramedics that had been linked to the clinic. It requested that state health department inspectors investigate. These enquiries supported the concerns.

On 28 April 2008, two dialysis patients reported that they saw Saenz injecting bleach from a cleaning bucket into the dialysis lines of patients (who later died). A dialysis line (IV or intravenous line) used in dialysis treatment comprises a soft plastic tube which is inserted into a large vein and connected to a dialysis machine. This enables blood to be circulated to the machine and back to the patient's body. Following the reported tampering, Saenz was sent home and was dismissed the next day. Police were called in and the clinic was temporarily closed.

Charged the following year, Saenz pleaded not guilty and was freed on bail. In 2012, she stood trial for the 2008 murders of five patients: Clara Strange, Thelma Metcalf, Garlin Kelley, Cora Bryant, and Opal Few. Defence lawyer Ryan Deaton argued that Saenz drew bleach into the syringes to ensure that she had the correct amount for the solutions that were used to disinfect the plastic lines. However, investigators having examined Saenz's computer testified that it revealed internet searches for bleach poisoning and its detection in dialysis lines.

Although Saenz had previously sworn an affidavit that she had no previous felony record, many anomalies emerged. There was evidence that she had overused prescription drugs, had addiction and substance abuse problems, had entered false information on a job application, and had been fired several times from healthcare jobs. Tried and found guilty in Texas District Court, Saenz was sentenced to life imprisonment without the possibility of parole (Graczyk/Associated Press 2015; Fox News, 31 March 2012).

Kimberly Clark Saenz—Analysis

Any attempts to **increase the effort** required by a perpetrator were effectively sidestepped because Kimberly Clark Saenz held a healthcare role.

Turning to **increasing the risks** to perpetrators, *extending guardianship* relates to authorities communicating concerns to future employers and others. Saenz was fired from Woodland Heights Hospital, Texas, for stealing drugs and had experienced problems of addiction and substance abuse. She had entered false information on a job application. Saenz had also sworn a false affidavit. Overall, she evaded strategies to filter out unsuitable employees. However, authorities acted to *assist natural surveillance* (whistle blowing) when dialysis patients reported seeing Saenz inject bleach into dialysis lines. Also, action was taken following an anonymous letter requesting an investigation into the clinic's high number of emergency calls for paramedics. Investigations acted to *strengthen formal surveillance* and confirmed suspicions.

Reducing rewards to the perpetrator and **reducing provocations** appear not to have arisen with Saenz.

Regarding **removing excuses**, an attempt to make excuses at Saenz's trial were successfully challenged. Defence lawyers suggested that Saenz used syringes for bleach to calibrate the amount when mixing the solutions used to disinfect the plastic lines. However, Saenz's computer showed internet searches for bleach poisoning.

Charles Cullen, US

Charles Cullen—The Case

Charles Cullen was born in West Orange, New Jersey, in 1960. At age 18 he enlisted in the navy, from which he was later medically discharged. He studied at nursing school in New Jersey from 1984, graduating three years later. Cullen then took a post at the burn unit of Saint Barnabas Medical Center, Livingston, New Jersey. In early 1992, the hospital discovered that intravenous bags were being contaminated. As the hospital began investigating this, Cullen left. (He confessed much later that he had killed several patients at Saint Barnabas Medical Center, including by intravenous drug overdose.) On leaving Saint Barnabas, Cullen moved to Warren Hospital, Phillipsburg, where he killed three elderly women patients with digitoxin overdoses.

His private life was unravelling. He and his wife divorced, and he moved to Phillipsburg. Cullen was arrested for stalking a female co-worker and given a year's probation. During this time, he attempted suicide and was treated for depression. In late 1993, Cullen left Warren Hospital.

From 1993 to 1996 Cullen worked at the intensive care unit of Hunterdon Medical Center, Flemington, where he murdered five patients with digitoxin overdoses. After a brief stint at Morristown Memorial Hospital, New Jersey, he was unemployed for several months. Cullen was briefly admitted to a psychiatric facility.

In early 1998, Cullen worked at the Liberty Nursing Home and Rehabilitation Center, Allentown, Pennsylvania. Accused of giving patients drugs outside scheduled times, he was eventually fired. He next moved to Easton Hospital, Pennsylvania, from November 1998 to March 1999, where he murdered a patient with digitoxin. Authorities were suspicious and investigated the death but lacked solid evidence.

Cullen then left Easton for Lehigh Valley Hospital, Allentown, where he killed a patient. In April 1999, he moved to St. Luke's Hospital in Bethlehem, Pennsylvania. There he killed five patients. In August 2000, a co-worker noticing Cullen hiding medication in bins used for needles reported this to hospital authorities. Pennsylvania State Police were called in but their investigation was inconclusive. In September 2002, Cullen worked at the Somerset Medical Center, Somerville, New Jersey, killing eight patients with digitoxin and other drugs. In mid-2003, Somerset Medical Center, having noticed irregularities in Cullen's performance, began investigating. Cullen was consulting records of patients to whom he was not assigned. He was erratic in his requests for patient drugs. Later that year, after a patient died from low blood sugar, the Center alerted state authorities. An investigation of Cullen's employment history revealed suspicions about his involvement in past deaths. The Medical Center fired Cullen and police put him under observation.

Finally, in December 2003, in Somerset, New Jersey detectives arrested Cullen for the murder of a patient at the Somerset Medical Center. Two days later Cullen confessed to killing, over 16 years, more than 30 patients. After several court hearings and guilty pleas, in 2006, Cullen was sentenced to multiple life sentences (Daily Mail Reporter 2013).

Charles Cullen—Analysis

Through his healthcare role, Cullen evaded strategies that might **increase the effort** required by a perpetrator.

With reference to **increasing the risks** to perpetrators, in several of Cullen's work settings, *natural surveillance* indicated something amiss. At Saint Barnabas Medical Center, New Jersey, it was noticed that intravenous bags were being contaminated but Cullen left as this was being investigated. A co-worker at St. Luke's Hospital, Pennsylvania, reported Cullen hiding medication, but a police investigation was inconclusive. *Formal surveillance* also alerted authorities. Cullen was fired from Liberty Nursing Home and Rehabilitation Center, Pennsylvania, accused of giving patients drugs at unscheduled times. Suspicious Easton Hospital authorities investigated a death but lacked clear evidence. Finally, Somerset Medical Center noticed Cullen inappropriately consulting patient records and making erratic drug requests. After a patient died and further suspicion was raised, investigations finally revealed the problems in Cullen's employment history. Opportunities for employers to *extending guardianship* were either missed by hospitals or evaded by Cullen. Authorities missed opportunities to communicate with other facilities. Also, facilities had not alerted other prospective employers to concerns. More generally Cullen's disturbed behaviour and known criminality were not systematically communicated with employers. Taken together such indications would have given pause to employers. Subsequently, Pennsylvania, New Jersey, and other states adopted laws protecting employers providing truthful and frank appraisals.

Authorities were unable to **reduce rewards** that Cullen presumably derived from his killings because he continually moved jobs before the consequences of his actions caught up with him. Similarly, techniques to **reduce provocations** did not arise because Cullen did not kill from any obvious provocation. Nor was it relevant to **remove excuses** because Cullen did not seek to excuse his actions.

Dr Harold Shipman, UK

Harold Shipman—The Case

Dr Harold Shipman (1946–2004) was the United Kingdom's most prolific serial killer. Married aged 19 he graduated medical school at 25 and worked in hospitals for several years. Entering general practice in 1974, he worked in Todmorden until 1979 when colleagues discovered that he had been dishonestly obtaining controlled drugs (pethidine) for his own use. Shipman pleaded guilty in court to drug charges. A year later, he became a General Practitioner at the Donnybrook practice in Hyde, near Manchester. Having left this practice in January 1992, Shipman worked as a sole practitioner in the same building. In October, he moved to a surgery nearby, again as a sole practitioner. For many he was a well-liked and respected physician.

From a practice in Hyde, in March 1998, Dr Linda Reynolds raised concerns with the South Manchester Coroner about the number of Shipman's patients who were dying and the circumstances. Greater Manchester Police conducted a confidential investigation, finding no substance in Dr Reynolds's concerns. On 17 April 1998, Shipman killed three more patients.

Shipman's patient Kathleen Grundy, aged 81, died at home in 1998. Her daughter, solicitor Angela Woodruff, was suspicious to find that her mother's will which she knew had left her estate to near relatives had been changed to favour Shipman shortly before Kathleen's death. Woodruff reported this and Greater Manchester Police searched Shipman's surgery and home. Kathleen's body was exhumed, revealing unexpectedly high levels of morphine. Police examined 19 deaths implicated in the investigation in March and further bodies were exhumed showing the presence of morphine. Examination of Shipman's computerised medical records showed tampering to hide the real cause of death by morphine. In April 1998, Shipman was arrested and charged with murder.

In 1999, Shipman pleaded 'not guilty' to 15 counts of murder. Found guilty on all counts, he was given a prison term of 15 life sentences. No further criminal proceedings were proposed, it being considered impossible for Shipman to receive a fair trial.

Between August 2000 and April 2001, inquests into 27 deaths of Shipman's patients were held. These recorded verdicts of unlawful killing in 25 and open verdicts in two. A month later, inquests into a further 232 deaths were opened, then immediately adjourned, pending the findings of a public enquiry. This enquiry was established in 2001, ultimately judging that Shipman murdered about 250 patients between 1971 and 1998, and positively determining 218. Typically, the method of killing was by a lethal dose of an opiate drug (usually diamorphine). Shipman committed suicide in prison in 2004 (Shipman Inquiry, December 2005).

Harold Shipman—Analysis

Any attempts to **increase the effort** of the perpetrator were inoperable because Shipman was inside the perimeter of safety precautions. As a physician, he had legitimate access to the morphine-based drugs that he misused to kill patients. Shipman subverted death certification procedures, dismissing any concerns expressed by relatives.

Regarding **increasing the risks** to the perpetrator, Shipman avoided *natural surveillance* by setting up as a sole practitioner, first in the same building as his previous Donnybrook practice, and later nearby. In 1998, Dr Reynolds raised concerns. However, when her natural surveillance was replaced by *formal surveillance* as police conducted confidential enquiries, investigators lacked the necessary expertise. Shipman's poisoning was ended through a combination of informal and formal surveillance as the solicitor daughter of one of Shipman's victims became suspicious that Shipman had forged her mother's will. This *formal surveillance/investigation* revealed Shipman's tampering with records of death on his computer.

Whatever **rewards** Shipman got from his killings they were unabated for decades. There were no obvious **provocations** to reduce. Neither did Shipman attempt to make **excuses** for his killings but pleaded not guilty and declined to cooperate with police.

Red Flags and Healthcare Serial Poisoners

One preventive approach to healthcare serial killers (including poisoners) is to study the personality and behaviour of known offenders, to try to identify potential causes for concern in current situations. Ramsland (2007) examined perpetrators' characteristics, motives, and methods and developed a 21-item 'red flag' checklist of features associated with healthcare serial killing. Some relate to behaviour, for example, 'Moves from one hospital to another' and 'Predicts when someone will die'. Other items describe aspects of personality such as 'History of mental instability/depression' or 'Appears to have a personality disorder'.

Building on this, Yardley and Wilson (2016) reviewed 16 cases of nurses convicted of serially killing patients and provide the percentage of cases in which each checklist item was noted. The highest scoring items in terms of the percentage of cases were 'Higher incidences of death on his/her shift' (94%), 'History of mental stability/depression' (63%), and 'Make colleagues anxious/suspicious' (56%).

Such checklists can raise awareness of behaviours and traits among healthcare workers that might compromise patient safety. But, the brevity of some items can be misleading. For example, 'Predicts when someone will die' could refer to a single occasion of anticipating a patient's impending death to alert relatives; or to persistent, accurate (and possibly suspicious) predictions of unexpected death. Unpacking what is intended might make the checklist unwieldy but more precise.

Some items suggest a fuller consideration. 'Prefers night shifts—fewer colleagues about' could raise broader questions (and perhaps a review) of night shift work such as staff preferences and their reasons, and the rigour of staff supervision in different shifts.

'Higher incidences of death on his/her shifts' suggest further careful enquiries. Among important considerations are the shifts being compared, the circumstances, the time scale, the exact definition of 'higher incidences', the statistical probabilities of differing death rates arising by chance, and the credibility of innocent explanations.

Such red flags can alert authorities to possible problems of patient safety requiring fuller investigation. Of even more direct concern is the findings of Yorker et al. (2006) that some convicted healthcare workers had falsified their credentials and/or fabricated critical events (such as sexual assault) before being suspected of murder. Yorker argues that healthcare employers should consider fraud or misrepresentation as a serious risk factor in patient safety. Caregivers' employment rights need to be balanced with the employers' need to know their employees' backgrounds. When a worker moves post, employers need to say if they were fired, or if their presence was associated with adverse patient outcomes. Authorities may fear negative publicity or retaliatory civil action but must fully cooperate with police enquiries and other investigations, or risk harm to patients (ibid.). At the same time, authorities need to avoid incorrectly accusing healthcare workers as happened with Nurse Daniela Poggiali in Italy (Day, 14 October 2014).

All this suggests being alert to possible red flags relating to the behaviour and personality of healthcare workers; and improving staff background checks, monitoring, and strategies for communicating concerns.

SCP Overview

Increase Perpetrators' Efforts

Tactics that might increase the effort required by a perpetrator were effectively sidestepped by Högel, Saenz, Cullen, and Shipman. Their healthcare role took each of them inside the safety perimeter that normally exists in healthcare facilities and services. Patients as *targets* were not *hardened* because suspicion was lacking. *Controlling access to facilities* and *screening exits* did not come into play because the perpetrators had legitimate access to facilities and patients. Similarly, *controlling tools/weapons* was evaded because the perpetrators had access to both medication and to patients.

Increase Perpetrators' Risks

Oldenburg authorities appear to have missed the opportunity to *extend guardianship*. Indeed, Högel was given a reference when he moved to Delmenhorst Hospital despite concerns about aspects of his behaviour.

With Saenz authorities failed to communicate information and concerns to future employers including being fired for stealing drugs, addiction problems, falsifying a job application, and swearing a false affidavit. In all this Saenz evaded any strategies to filtering out unsuitable employees. Regarding Cullen, either hospitals missed opportunities to extend their guardianship or Cullen evaded them. Authorities missed opportunities to communicate concerns with other facilities. State laws were passed to try to improve matters but after the event.

Turning to *assisting natural surveillance*, with Högel any natural surveillance seems to have been insufficiently backed up, missing the implications of his keenness to show off his resuscitation skills, and increased death rates. Authorities responded to whistle blowing when dialysis patients reported seeing **Saenz** injecting bleach into dialysis lines and followed up an anonymous letter raising concerns. In several settings where Cullen worked, natural surveillance indicated problems. However, when authorities noticed that intravenous bags were being contaminated and began investigating, Cullen left; and when a co-worker reported Cullen hiding medication, police investigations were inconclusive. Shipman limited the opportunities for others to exercise natural surveillance by becoming a sole practitioner. Despite this, Dr Reynolds exercised good natural surveillance when she raised concerns.

Regarding Saenz, investigations acted to *strengthen formal surveillance* and showed that emergency crews had been called excessively. With Högel formal surveillance was not strong enough to detect warning signs and lead to decisive action. However, formal surveillance led to Cullen being fired from Liberty Nursing Home and Rehabilitation Center, Pennsylvania, and precipitated an investigation at Easton Hospital, Pennsylvania (although clear evidence was lacking). Also, Somerset Medical Center noticed Cullen inappropriately consulting patient records and making erratic requests for patient drugs leading to further suspicions and action. With Shipman, formal surveillance, when police conducted confidential enquiries, was impaired by investigators' lack of expertise. But his demise came when police were alerted about suspicions that he had forged a patient's Will.

Reduce Perpetrators' Rewards

Reducing rewards to the perpetrator appears not to have been relevant with Högel, Saenz, Cullen, and Shipman because there was often insufficient suspicion of anything amiss. Also, perpetrators actively evaded scrutiny.

Reduce Provocations

With healthcare serial poisoners, authorities seek to *discourage imitation*. They try to balance revealing modus operandi which might encourage imitation, and publicising offenses to alert other authorities. When Högel was apprehended authorities seemingly judged that the publicity would discourage imitation rather than encourage other potential healthcare serial poisoners. It would also alert hospitals to the risks of such perpetrators.

Remove Excuses

Removing excuses for example by 'alerting conscience' does not seem to arise routinely with healthcare serial poisoners. Högel made no excuses for his killings but used them as a scenario for his self-aggrandisement. Cullen sought no excuse for his actions. Neither did Shipman attempt to excuse his killings but pleaded not guilty and declined to cooperate with police. An attempt to make excuses at Saenz's trial was removed. Claims that she used syringes for bleach to calibrate the amount needed to disinfect the plastic lines were undermined when Saenz's computer showed internet searches for bleach poisoning.

Means, Motive, Opportunity, Location, and Perpetrator-Victim Relationship

Means

In some cases, nursing specialisms inform the exact means that perpetrators use to offend. Nurses look after patients with heart problems, respiratory difficulties, and diabetes where drug regimens help to stabilise patients' health. Murder by interfering with the correct drug doses can create signs and symptoms similar to those of the patient's illness, for example, cardiac problems.

Högel used overdoses of ajmaline, sotalol, lidocaine/xylocaine, amiodarone, and potassium chloride which can precipitate potentially fatal cardiac arrhythmia and lowered blood pressure. Cullen killed patients with digitoxin overdoses. Shipman typically murdered patients with a fatal opiate dose (usually diamorphine) before falsifying the cause of death and his patients' records. On a different tack, Saenz injected bleach from a cleaning bucket into the dialysis lines of patients, claiming it was part of a disinfecting procedure.

Motive

Motives of healthcare serial poisoners include seeking excitement and self-aggrandisement, sadistic satisfaction, and unjustifiably claimed mercy killing. Among rare motives are financial gain, jealousy, and revenge (Farrell 2018, pp. 100–107). Högel referred in court to seeking the excitement of unpredictability—elated when able to resuscitate a patient and dejected otherwise. Each time a patient died he would unsuccessfully promise to himself not to repeat the game. Saenz's motives are unclear, but her killings were intentional, and her work background included malign behaviour and deception. Although his exact motives for killing are unknown, Cullen showed disturbed behaviour and criminality over long periods. Speculation about why Shipman committed his crimes include that he had a warped sense of serving society by reducing the burden on the health system. Alternatively, he may have gained satisfaction from being the arbiter of life and death. But his motives essentially remain unknown.

Opportunity

Opportunity for killing arises through the healthcare role. A perpetrator has intimate contact with vulnerable clients, access to drugs and knowledge of their action, the trust of the community, knowledge of the routines of medical facilities, and understanding of how medical services work. Seizing such opportunities was evident with Högel and Cullen, to a lesser extent with Saenz (whose medical knowledge was limited), and to a remarkable degree with Shipman.

Location

Högel murdered victims at the Oldenburg Clinic and later at Delmenhorst. Saenz killed patients at a dialysis clinic in Lufkin. Cullen murdered at several medical centres and hospitals in New Jersey and Pennsylvania, changing workplace if suspicions were aroused. Shipman's victims were patients from the geographical areas of his practices, usually killed on home visits when alone, and willing to accept injections as part of their treatment.

Perpetrator-Victim Relationship

Högel's victims were judged to be around 36 patients at the Oldenburg Clinic, and 48 patients at Delmenhorst. Some estimates put the figure considerably higher. It is reported that Högel's victims were aged from 34 to 96 years (Laws 2019). Saenz was charged with the murders of five patients: Clara Strange, Thelma Metcalf, Garlin Kelley, Cora Bryant, and Opal Few. Cullen confessed to killing more than 30 patients over a period of 16 years. There is much detail of Shipman's victims because a judge-led enquiry sought to identify them all. Although the youngest was 41-year-old Peter Lewis and the oldest 93-year-old Ann Cooper, victims were mostly in their 70s, 80s, and 90s. Often relatives might be expecting their deaths because of age or illness. About four times as many women as men were victims—perhaps reflecting their greater preponderance among elderly populations. There appeared to be no selection of victims according to any social, occupational, or ethnic pattern.

Conclusion

Red Flags and Healthcare Serial Poisoners

Research indicates that among indicators of potential concern are employees who have a history of mental instability/depression, who make colleagues anxious/suspicious, and on whose shifts there are more deaths (Ramsland 2007; Yardley and Wilson 2016). Issues raised by checklists may require fuller investigation. Yorker et al. (2006) found that some convicted healthcare workers falsified their credentials or fabricated critical events (or both) before being suspected of murder. Yorker argues that healthcare employers should consider fraud or misrepresentation as a serious risk factor in patient safety. Caregivers' employment rights need to be balanced with the employers' need to know their employees' backgrounds. This suggests being alert to possible red flags relating to the behaviour and personality of healthcare workers and improving staff background checks, monitoring, and strategies for communicating concerns.

Situational Crime Prevention and Healthcare Serial Poisoners

Attempts to *harden targets, control access to facilities, screen exits, deflect offenders*, and *control tools/weapons* can be sidestepped. The healthcare role takes perpetrators inside the safety perimeter of healthcare facilities and services.

Failures to *extend guardianship* occur where authorities provide positive employee references despite concerns, or otherwise fail to communicate suspicions to new employers. Employers may not be rigorous enough in checking their employees past records, criminal convictions, misconduct, psychiatric treatment, and false claims. Any *natural surveillance* reflected by staff expressing concerns may not always be supported by employers. Where whistle blowing is acted upon, authorities can expedite investigations and may save lives. Perpetrators can sometimes evade the consequences of surveillance by leaving an employment or isolating themselves as a sole practitioner. *Formal surveillance* may be too weak to detect concerns and produce decisive action. Checks for irregularities including in staff members issuing medication may be ineffective. Where such checks are efficient, they can lead to further investigation and preventive action.

Efforts to *conceal targets, remove targets, identify property, disrupt markets,* and *deny benefits* can be rendered ineffective if there is insufficient suspicion of anything amiss. Also, perpetrators can evade scrutiny by changing employer.

Attempts to *reduce frustrations and stress, avoid disputes, reduce emotional arousal,* and *neutralise peer pressure* do not typically apply with healthcare serial poisoners. To *discourage imitation* authorities try to limit revealing modus operandi which might encourage imitation, while publicising offenses to alert medical facilities and others.

Removing excuses does not arise routinely with healthcare serial poisoners who tend not to make excuses for their actions. Where excuses are made, they can be challenged if there is evidence that the perpetrator intended to harm patients.

Means, Motive, Opportunity, Location, and Perpetrator-Victim Relationship

Means of poisoning patients are typically through overdoses of medication. Nursing duties include looking after patients with conditions where lethal overdoses of treatment drugs can create signs and symptoms like those of the patient's illness.

Healthcare serial poisoners' motives have included seeking excitement and self-aggrandisement, sadistic satisfaction, unjustifiably claimed mercy killing, and more rarely financial gain, jealousy, and revenge (Farrell 2018, pp. 100–107). Poisoners may seek the thrill of intervening to rescue patients from the jeopardy they have created. They may have the warped notion that they are reducing the health burden on society. Sometimes poisoners' motives are unknown or unclear.

Opportunity for killing arises from the healthcare worker role (intimate contact with vulnerable clients, trust of the community, access to drugs and knowledge of their action, understanding of how medical services work, and knowledge of the routines of medical facilities).

Regarding healthcare serial poisoners, the location of murder is predictably the medical facility at which workers are employed. Frequent changes of workplace can conceal wrongdoing. Murder may take place on medical home visits where the patient is alone and unsupervised.

The relationship between a healthcare serial poisoner and their victims is typically (and by definition) that of patient and medical practitioner. This relationship provides victims and protects the perpetrator from suspicion, allowing the sometimes disturbingly high numbers of victims. Often victims are ill (but may be recovering) and may be elderly. Victims do not appear to be selected according to any social, occupational, or ethnic pattern.

Suggested Activities

Select a recent case of healthcare serial poisoning from your own country or elsewhere. Gather information to give as clear a picture as possible of what happened. Reviewing the red flag approach, which aspects might have been the strongest preventive ones? Which aspects of SCP might have helped prevent the killings?

Key Text

Yardley, E., & Wilson, D. (2016). In Search of the 'Angels of Death': Conceptualising the Contemporary Nurse Healthcare Serial Killer. *Journal of Investigative Psychology and Offender Profiling, 13*(1), 39–55.

Building on a red flag approach this article reviews cases of nurses convicted of serially killing patients and identifies the percentage of cases in which specific items were noted.

References

Associated Press. (1990, January 25). Nurse Gets 50 Years to Life. *Times Daily*.

Associated Press. (2006, October 3). Life Term for Ex-nurse in Patient Killings. *NBC News*. Retrieved from http://www.nbcnews.com/id/15119953/ns/us_news-crime_and_courts/t/life-term-ex-nurse-patient-killings/#. WgwGcWi0OM8.

Behavioural Analysis Unit. (2005). *Serial Murders: Multi-disciplinary Perspectives for Investigators*. Washington, DC: National Center for the Analysis of Violent Crime, US Department of Justice.

Bryant, E. (2003, January 31). Nurse Sentenced for Killing Patients. *United Press International*. Retrieved from www.upi.com/Business_News/Security-Industry/2003/01/31/Nurse-sentenced-for-killing-patients/UPI-96721044036550/.

Campbell, D. (2011, October 4). 'Angel of Death' Colin Norris Could Be Cleared of Insulin Murders. *The Guardian*.

Cleaver, H. (2006, February 8). Angel of Death 'Driven by Kindness'. *The Telegraph*.

Connell, R. (2011, March 28). Dorothea Puente Dies at 82: Boarding House Operator Who Killed Tenants. *Los Angeles Times*.

Daily Mail Reporter. (2013, April 29). 'Angel of Death' Nurse Who Murdered at Least 40 Patients to Become One of America's Worst Serial Killers Speaks from Prison for the First Time to Chillingly Claim: 'I Thought I Was Helping'. *Mail Online*.

Day, M. (2014, October 14). Italian Nurse Daniela Poggiali Is Accused of Killing 'Up to 38 Patients Because She Found Them Annoying'. *The Independent*. Retrieved from http://www.independent.co.uk/news/world/europe/italian-nurse-under-investigation-for-killing-up-to-38-patients-because-she-found-them-annoying-9793181.html.

DW News Report. (2019). Retrieved from https://allthatsinteresting.com/niels-hogel.

Eddy, M. (2019, May 10). Hundreds of Bodies, One Nurse: German Serial Killer Leaves as Many Questions as Victims. *New York Times*.

Ephemeral New York. (2015). Serial Killer Frederick Mors. Retrieved from https://ephemeralnewyork.wordpress.com/tag/serial-killer-frederick-mors/.

Farragher, T. (2000, October 8). Death on Ward C _ Caregiver Or Killer. *The Boston Globe Online*. Retrieved from http://cache.boston.com/globe/metro/packages/nurse/part1.htm.

Farrell, M. (2018). *Criminology of Serial Poisoners*. London: Palgrave Macmillan.

Fox News. (2012, March 31). Texas Nurse Convicted in Bleach Deaths Case. Retrieved from http://www.foxnews.com/us/2012/03/31/texas-nurse-convicted-in-bleach-deaths-case.html.

Glaister, J. (1954). *The Power of Poison*. London: C. Johnson.

Graczyk, M., & Associated Press. (2015, November 14). Nurse's Bleach Injection Deaths Trial Begins. KIMATV. Retrieved from http://kimatv.com/news/nation-world/nurses-bleach-injection-deaths-trial-begins-11-14-2015-230029540.

Hickey, E. (2010). *Serial Murderers and Their Victims* (5th ed.). Belmont, CA: Wadsorth.

Holmes, R. M., & Holmes, S. T. (2010). *Serial Murder* (3rd ed.). London: Sage.

Kinnell, H. G. (2000). Serial Homicide by Doctors: Shipman in Perspective. *British Medical Journal, 321*, 1594–1597.

Laws, J. (2019, May 16). 'Angel of Death' German Nurse 42 Who Killed 97 Hospital Patients Should Face Life in Jail Say Prosecutors. *Mail On Line and APF*.

Lieberman, P. (2002, April 18). Hospital 'Angle of Death' Gets Life Without Parole. *Los Angeles Times*. Retrieved from http://articles.latimes.com/2002/apr/18/news/mn-38536.

Maeder, T. (1980). *The Unspeakable Crimes of Dr Petiot*. Boston, MA: Little Brown.

McQuigge, M, (2017, June 2). If You Ever Do This Again, We'll Turn You in Pastor Tells Killer Nurse. *The Canadian Press*. Retrieved from www.thestar.com/news/canada/2017/06/02/if-you-ever-do-this-again-well-turn-you-in-pastor-told-killer-nurse.html.

Oltermann, P. (2017, August 28). German Nurse Suspected of Murdering at Least 90 Patients. *The Guardian*. Retrieved from www.theguardian.com/world/2017/aug/28/german-nurse-niels-hoegel-suspected-murdering-90-patients.

Payne, S. (2006, April 19). Guilty of Murder: The Nurse Who Got His Kicks from Life-or-Death Drama. *The Telegraph*.

Ramsland, K. (2007). *Inside the Minds of Healthcare Serial Killers: Why They Kill*. Westport, CT: Praeger.

Reporter. (1884, May 11). Marie Jeanneret's Death-Grim Facts in the Career of This Famous Poisoner. *New York Times*, p. 5. (Reprinted from *The London Daily News*).

Reporter. (1902, July 27). Poison Her Passion. *The Clinton Morning Age*. Retrieved from www.news.google.com/newspapers?nid=2267&dat=190207 27&id=6ncmAAAAIBAJ&sjid=CgEGAAAAIBAJ&pg=4194,9968 21&hl=en.

Reporter. (1992, April 10, Friday). Nurse Pleads Guilty to Killing Three Patients. *New York Times*. Retrieved from www.nytimes.com/1992/04/10/us/nurse-pleads-guilty-to-killing-three-patients.html.

Scheerhout, J. (2015). Did Killer Nurse Victorina Chua Pay Someone to Pass His Nursing Exam? *Manchester Evening News*. Updated 18 May 2015.

Shipman Inquiry. (2005, December). Fifth Report *Safeguarding Patients: Lessons from the Part – Proposals for the Future*. Retrieved from http://webarchive. nationalarchives.gov.uk/20090808154959/http://www.the-shipman-inquiry.org.uk/fr_page.asp.

Stewart, J. B. (1999). *Blind Eye: How the Medical Establishment Let a Doctor Get Away with Murder*. New York: Simon and Schuster.

Trestrail, J. H. (2007). *Criminal Poisoning: Investigational Guide for Law Enforcement, Toxicologists, Forensic Scientists and Attorneys* (2nd ed.). Totowa, NJ: Humana Press.

United Press International. (1986, March 31). Suspected Nurse Had History of Mental Illness. *Orlando Sentinel*.

Wilson, C., & Seaman, D. (1983). *Encyclopaedia of Modern Murder: 1962–1982*. London: Barker.

Yardley, E., & Wilson, D. (2016). In Search of the 'Angels of Death': Conceptualising the Contemporary Nurse Healthcare Serial Killer. *Journal of Investigative Psychology and Offender Profiling, 13*(1), 39–55.

Yorker, B. C., Kizer, K. W., Lampe, P., Forest, A. R. W., Lannan, J. M., & Russell, D. A. (2006). Serial Murder by Healthcare Professionals. *Journal of Forensic Science, 51*(6), 1–10.

4

Assassination and Poisoning

Introduction

Dramatic examples of political assassinations and plots involving poison have occurred in recent years. Sergei and Yulia Skripal were poisoned with Novichok in Salisbury, England, in March 2018. In February 2017 Kim Jong-nam, half-brother of the North Korean leader Kim Jong-un, was poisoned at Kuala Lumpur airport, Malaysia, with a chemical liquid. Russian spy Alexander Litvinenko, a political exile in the United Kingdom, died in November 2006, poisoned by polonium-210. Bulgarian dissident writer Georgi Markov died in 1978 from ricin poisoning, implicating the Bulgarian Secret Service. The chapter considers these attacks in relation to Situational Crime Prevention (SCP) and to the issues of means, motive, opportunity, location, and perpetrator-victim relationships.

© The Author(s) 2020
M. Farrell, *Criminology of Poisoning Contexts*,
https://doi.org/10.1007/978-3-030-40830-5_4

Defining and Classifying Assassination

Materials relating to a 1954 CIA operation in Guatemala (code named PBSUCCESS) included CIA training files with a guidebook on political killing, describing the procedures, instruments, and conduct of assassinations (CIA Manual c1954). Assassination was categorised according to the subject, the assassin, and whether there was concealment or publicity. A subject might be unaware of being targeted ('simple'); aware but unguarded ('chase'); or aware and protected ('guarded'). An assassin could plan to die with the subject ('lost') or to escape ('safe'). Concealment could be necessary ('secret'), or immaterial ('open'), or publicity could be required ('terroristic') (ibid.). Killers may use: the hands or improvised weapons, drugs including medical overdoses and poisons, explosives, firearms, or 'edge weapons' such as knives. Death may be made to appear accidental such as a fall from a high building (ibid.).

As we will see later, the poisonings of Skripal, Kim Jong-un, Litvinenko, and Markov were 'chase' and 'safe'. They were partly 'terroristic' in that they were intended to spread fear among defectors but not necessarily among the wider public. All the victims were unguarded, but likely aware of being a potential target. All the perpetrators envisaged their escape. In the Skripal attempt, the poison was deposited to contaminate the victims after the attackers had gone. In killing Kim Jong-nam the planners escaped, leaving the direct perpetrators to be detained. With Litvinenko and Markov, slow-acting poison allowed the attackers to get away. In all instances poisoning was intended to eliminate defectors or critics of their country, while deterring others.

Poison Assassinations in Recent History

Poison has figured in assassinations and plots associated with Cold War tensions and unwelcome nationalist trends. In 1953 in Vienna, Soviet assassin Iosif Grigulevich and his controllers discussed plans to kill President Tito of Yugoslavia. Schemes included infecting the leader in a face-to-face meeting with pulmonary plague bacteria dispensed by an assassin protected by an antidote. Alternatively, a stooge would present Tito with a gift box which when opened would release poison gas killing everyone present (Wise and Ross 1967).

Ukrainian Bogdan Stashynsky was recruited and trained by the KGB. In 1957, in Munich, he assassinated Ukrainian nationalist leader and political exile Dr Lev Rebet, using a concealed tubular gun that vaporised a lethal poison. Before the assassination, the killer took an antidote pill, afterwards inhaling a further antidote from an ampoule (Anders 1967, pp. 9–39). In Munich in 1959 using a similar weapon Stashynsky assassinated Stefan Bandera, another Ukrainian nationalist leader (ibid., pp. 41–55).

Anti-colonialist Cameroon leader Félix-Roland Moumié was assassinated in Geneva in 1960. The killer who escaped was likely a former agent of the SDECE, the French Intelligence Service. Poisoned with thallium, Moumié died some weeks later (Tchouteu 2017).

Following the independence of the Republic of Congo from Belgian rule, Katangan secessionists opposed the government of Prime Minister Patrice Lumumba. As Lumumba turned to the Soviet Union for help, the CIA prepared poison for an agent to take to Africa to kill him. Before this transpired, in 1961, Lumumba was deposed and assassinated by a firing squad commanded by members of the Belgium-backed Katangan forces (De Witte [1999]/2002).

A report by the CIA Inspector General in May 1967 outlined plots to kill Cuba's President Castro. Schemes included using a pen syringe with a fine needle to introduce a poison undetected, and giving Castro a contaminated skin-diving suit (Escalante, [commentary] 2008). Poison assassinations and plots continue to the present day. It is to these more recent events that we now turn.

Situational Crime Prevention

SCP is fully described in Chap. 2. Briefly, five general strategies are each associated with five opportunity reducing techniques. Techniques to **increase the effort** of perpetrators are 'target harden', 'control access to facilities', 'screen exits', 'deflect offenders', and 'control tools/weapons'.

Increase the risks concerns 'extend guardianship', 'assist natural surveillance', 'reduce anonymity', 'utilise place managers', and 'strengthen formal surveillance'. Techniques to **reduce rewards** to the perpetrator are 'conceal targets', 'remove targets', 'identify property', 'disrupt markets', and 'deny benefits'. **Reduce provocations** involves 'reduce frustrations and stress', 'avoid disputes', 'reduce emotional arousal', 'neutralise peer pressure', and 'discourage imitation'. **Remove excuses** concerns 'set rules', 'post instructions', 'alert conscience', 'assist compliance', and 'control drugs and alcohol'.

Sergei and Yulia Skripal

Skripal—The Poisoning

Born in Kaliningrad in 1951, Sergei Skripal studied at the Zhdanov Higher Military Engineering School, later joining the elite Russian Airborne Troops. He attended the Military Diplomatic Academy, Moscow, the secret training college of the GRU (foreign military intelligence agency). For five years Skripal was an attaché in Malta. In 1993, stationed in Madrid, he was recruited by MI5 as a double agent for the British. Retiring from GRU activities in 1997, he worked with Russian local officials. In 2004, Skripal was imprisoned for treason, but freed early under a Moscow-Washington spy swap. In 2010 Skripal moved to England, settling in Salisbury, with his wife Lyudmila, who died two years later.

Yulia Skripal, 33, Sergei and Lyudmila's daughter, graduated from Moscow State Humanities University in 2008 and then worked for Nike. In 2010 she followed Sergio to England and worked organising hotel conferences. In 2014 Yulia returned to Moscow. (Urban 2018).

In March 2018, Yulia visited her father in Salisbury. On Sunday, 4 March, at 4.15 pm the pair were seen gravely ill on a public bench in the city centre. Both were admitted to Salisbury District Hospital. Detective Sergeant Bailey, sent to investigate Sergei Skripal's house, became ill and was hospitalised. Poisoning was suspected. Samples of a substance found on Skripal's house door were identified as Novichok by the Defence Chemical Biological Radiological and Nuclear Centre, Porton Down, Wiltshire. Counter-terrorism police and military personnel became involved (Harley and Sawer 2018). Investigators believed that the poison was applied on Skripal's door on the morning of Sunday, 4 March, while father and daughter visited the local cemetery, returning around 1 pm. Both survived and, discharged from hospital in spring 2018, were moved to a secure location. Detective Sergeant Bailey also recovered.

In June 2018, Salisbury residents Charley Rowley, 45, and his partner Dawn Sturgess, 44, living on the fringes of society, found an apparent perfume bottle while scouring rubbish. At Rowley's house, Sturgess applied some of the 'perfume', fell ill, and died on 8 July. Having barely touched the poison, Rowley became poorly but survived (Urban 2018, p. 296).

In September 2018, UK authorities accused two men, believed to be Russian agents, of the Skripal attack, Alexander Petrov and Ruslan Boshirov, presumably aliases. Seeking the perpetrators' real identity, the investigative website Bellingcat worked with Russian partners 'The Insider', and Russian journalists visited the suspects' home villages. St Petersburg investigative website 'Fontanka' also contributed (Mark Urban, private communication, February 2019).

Bellingcat claimed that 'Boshirov' was a GRU colonel Anatoly Chepiga. Born in 1979 in Nikolaevka, Chepiga later entered the Far-Eastern Military Command Academy graduating from the military school in 2001. By 2010 he worked in Moscow as a clandestine GRU officer (Bellingcat Investigation Team, 26 September 2018a). 'Petrov' was GRU member Dr Alexander Mishkin. Born in 1979 in Loyga, Mishkin trained as a physician for the Russian naval armed forces before joining the GRU (ibid., 9 October 2018b).

Chepiga and Mishkin travelled from Moscow to Gatwick airport, England, on 2 March 2018. Next day they visited Salisbury for reconnaissance, before contaminating the Skripal door using a modified perfume bottle spray on Sunday, 4 March. That night they flew from Heathrow airport to Moscow (BBC, 8 October 2018). Following the incident, the United Kingdom and other countries expelled over 150 Russian diplomats. Russian authorities denied involvement and expelled foreign diplomats in retaliation. In 2018 the suspects told Russian broad-caster RT that they visited Salisbury as tourists (BBC, 8 October 2018). In January 2019, a Kremlin spokesman insisted that the men were 'sus-pected groundlessly' (Emmott and Balmforth 2019).

Skripal—Analysis

Regarding **increasing the effort** of perpetrators Sergio Skripal and Yulia were not sufficiently *hardened* as *targets* by the intelligence services to prevent an attack. Following the poisoning, police and media provided warnings to safeguard the public as secondary targets. While generally effective, these precautions could not avert Dawn Sturgess's unpredict-able death. *Controlling weapons* (poison) was ineffective because despite domestic legal restrictions on the sale and distribution of poison, the Novichok appears to have been smuggled into the United Kingdom.

Turning to **increasing risks** to perpetrators, the international expul-sion of Russian diplomats aimed to remind Russia of the *increased risk* of attempting assassination. Following the Salisbury attack, members of the public were alerted to carry out *natural surveillance* while authorities stepped up *formal surveillance*. This helped protect the public from fur-ther contact with the nerve agent that had spread beyond the Skripal house. But by this time the perpetrators had returned to Russia.

With reference to **reducing rewards** to the perpetrator, Sergio Skripal was not *concealed as a target* from the would-be assassins. However, after the attack father and daughter were *removed* to secret location. Attackers were *denied the benefits* of success because the Skripals' lives were saved.

The provocation to Russia was that Sergio Skripal had been a spy and British efforts to **reduce provocation** involved international diplomatic reprisals aimed at *discouraging imitation* of the assassination.

Concerning **removing excuses**, Russian denials of involvement in the Skripal incident were effectively *removed* by police investigations, enqui-ries by other authorities, and the work of Bellingcat and its associates. CCTV evidence was produced, and information about the identities of the suspects was distributed.

Kim Jong-nam

Kim Jong-nam: The Poisoning

Kim Jong-nam was born in 1971, in Pyongyang. He was the eldest son of Kim Jong-il who became leader of North Korea in 1994, his mother being one of three women with whom Kim Jong-il had children. Kim Jong-nam was first home-tutored by an aunt, then attended international schools in Switzerland and Russia. Returning to North Korea in 1988, he attended university in Pyongyang (Lee 2003).

Kim Jong-nam was expected to assume leadership of North Korea should Kim Jong-il die but fell from favour in the early 2000s. Exiled in 2003, and living in Macau, China, and elsewhere he continued to criticise the North Korean regime (Watts and Branigan 2012). Kim Jong-nam's paternal half-brother Kim Jong-un was nominated heir apparent in 2010, and, when the leader died a year later, assumed power.

On 13 February 2017, Kim Jong-nam was passing through Kuala Lumpur International Airport, Malaysia. At around 9 am in the departure hall, two women approached him. Soon afterwards, he told an airport receptionist that a woman had covered his face with a wet cloth and that he felt unwell. Treated at the Menara Medical Clinic and then stretchered to an ambulance for transfer to Putrajaya Hospital, Kim Jong-nam died en route to hospital. He was 45 years old. An autopsy at the KL Hospital mortuary indicated poisoning. Later, the Malaysian police chief announced that toxicologists had identified traces of the nerve agent VX on Kim's face.

On 14 February, Malaysian police arrested suspect Doan Thi Huong, identified from airport CCTV footage. Two days later, a second suspect Siti Aisyah was arrested. Huong told police that four male fellow travellers had persuaded her as a prank to spray Kim with an unknown liquid while Aisyah covered his face with a handkerchief. (This is conversant with using 'binary' chemicals that are individually non-lethal but combine to constitute poison such as VX.) Huong stated that the others having disappeared, she returned to the airport the following day when she was arrested.

According to Malaysian police Doan Thi Huong, a 28-year-old Vietnamese woman, worked in an entertainment outlet. Her family laboured on a rice farm in Northern Vietnam (Foreign Staff, February 2017). Siti Aisyah, a 25-year-old Indonesian woman from Serang, west of Jakarta, had two conflicting sets of identity papers. In one, she is born in 1992 and is an entrepreneur. In the second (naming her as Siti Aisah) she is a housewife born in 1989. Formerly a domestic help in Jakarta, she moved to Malaysia with her husband and their young son. She subsequently divorced and worked in a Kuala Lumpur night club (Babulal 2017).

Brought to trial in Selangor, Malaysia, on 2 October 2017, both women pleaded not guilty. Prosecution lawyers alleged that the two women together, and acting with four North Korean male fugitives, assassinated Kim Jong-nam. Having been recruited by North Korean operatives, the two women were trained as assassins to use VX.

Defence lawyers argued that the accused believed that they were acting in a prank reality television programme, unaware that they were using poison (Daily Excelsior 2019). In March 2019, the prosecutor successfully requested that the murder charge against Siti Aisyah be dropped and she was released. It was speculated that there was less evidence against Siti Aisyah than against her co-defendant (BBC News, 11 March 2019). A month later the defence lawyer for Doan Thi Huong announced that she had pleaded guilty to a lesser charge of causing harm and would be released. Four North Korean men wanted in connection with the murder are still at large (Sky News/www.youtube.com/watch?v=D_BN3y-ozqc).

On the political front, the South Korean government accused its northern neighbour of being responsible for the assassination, while the US Department of State claimed that North Korean operatives had used VX nerve gas. North Korean government officials denied that Kim Jong-nam had been assassinated, stating that he had died of a heart attack.

Kim Jong-nam: Analysis

For increasing the effort of perpetrators, any security precautions seeking to make Kim Jong-nam a *hard target* were ineffective. If the two women attackers were set up, their organisers escaped because they did not attract suspicion and evaded the routine procedures for *controlling access and exit* at airports. Procedures to *control weapons* in airports were seemingly circumvented by using binary chemicals.

Increasing the risks to perpetrators in the Malaysian killing involved CCTV *formal surveillance* which helped identify the women attackers. Kim Jong-nam also alerted staff who formed part of the airport's general *natural surveillance* and awareness.

Concerning **reducing rewards** to the perpetrator Kim Jong-nam was not sufficiently *concealed as a target* to evade assassination. The attack occurred in a public, yet designated, space where extra private security precautions may have been considered less essential.

Turning to **reducing provocations**, Kim Jong-nam may have been assassinated because of perceived political *provocation* against North Korea. Publishing (restricted) details of the perpetrators and the modus operandi sought to *discourage imitation* and indicate that such attacks can be identified. However, if the accused women were duped and the core perpetrators escaped, such a deterrent was toothless.

Concerning **removing excuses**, the North Korean claim that Kim Jong-nam died of a heart attack was countered by toxicological evidence implicating a nerve agent.

Alexander Litvinenko

Litvinenko: The Poisoning

Alexander Litvinenko was born in Voronezh, Russia, in 1962. After joining the army, he eventually became a KGB officer. In 1991 following the demise of the Union of Soviet Socialist Republics, the KGB morphed into the Federal Security Service (FSB). Litvinenko's work included investigating Russia's criminal underworld and, after publicising their links with the FSB, he was imprisoned for several months. In November 2000 Litvinenko, his wife and son vacationed in Turkey. On return transit to Moscow via London they defected (Goldfarb and Litvinenko 2007, pp. 3–19).

Billionaire Boris Berezovsky, whose life Litvinenko had saved in Russia by uncovering a plot to kill him, also defected to London. In 2003, Berezovsky bought a London house which he rented to Litvinenko to whom he paid a monthly salary. Litvinenko's work included publishing material damaging to President Putin, which led to a book accusing the FSB of being behind several Moscow bombings in 1999 (Litvinenko and Felshstinsky 2007). At the time, Chechen rebels were accused and the Kremlin ordered attacks on the breakaway republic. Reportedly, in the two years before his death, Litvinenko worked undercover for MI6, the British secret intelligence service (Harding 2015). Litvinenko also prepared due diligence reports on Russian individuals and companies (Owen 2016, sections 10.1 to 10.3).

In 2006, Litvinenko, now a British citizen, lived with his family in Muswell Hill, London. On the evening of Wednesday, 1 November 2006, he fell ill. Admitted to Barnet General Hospital on 3 November, he was later transferred to University College Hospital, London. His condition declined and on 23 November he died, aged 44. Litvinenko's illness was mysterious until shortly before his death when test results returned from the Atomic Weapons Establishment, Aldermaston. Samples of the patient's blood and urine indicated high levels of polonium-210, a radioactive isotope. This poison had caused lethal acute radiation syndrome (Owen 2016, sections 10.4 to 10.6).

On the afternoon of 1 November 2006 (the day that he became ill) Litvinenko had met two Russian men in the Pine bar of the Millennium Hotel, London. Andrei Lugovoi, 40, was a former KGB officer. He had met Litvinenko for the first time when after his KGB service he became head of security at a television channel ORT owned by Boris Berezovsky. Lugovoi's associate, Dmitry Kovtun, 40, had attended the Soviet Military Command Academy in the 1980s. The men joined Litvinenko for tea when one or both poisoned his drink with liquid polonium-210. Earlier, on 16 October 2006, the men had attempted to poison Litvinenko at a meeting at Erinys International, a security company (Owen 2016, sections 10.6 to 10.13). A third man Vladislav Sokolenko also attended the Millennium Hotel meeting (Cobain et al. 2006).

Polonium-210 must be produced and deployed to be harmless to the assassin, suggesting substantial resources and organisation behind the killing. An enquiry into Litvinenko's death reported that the assassins were 'probably' under the direction of the FSB whose operation was 'probably' approved by Russian spy chief Nikolai Patrushev and by President Putin (Owen 2016, sections 10.15 to 10.16). Dunkerley (2016) criticises the report for insufficiently recognising a 'misinformation campaign' led by Putin critic Berezovsky that Putin was culpable, and for using inconsistent standards of evidence. Putin disclaimed knowledge of the killing. Russian official Viktor Ivanov dismissed the *Litvinenko Report* (Reporter 2016 *Irish Times*). Sixsmith (2007) concludes that Litvinenko was killed by a group within the FSB working independently of the Kremlin to revenge the betrayal of their previous colleagues.

When Scotland Yard detectives interviewed Lugovoi and Kovtun in Moscow, the men claimed innocence, stating that they too had been poisoned. In August 2007, Lugovoi told London journalists via video link from Russia that both MI6 and Berezovsky were involved in Litvinenko's death (Emsley 2008, pp. 212–213).

Litvinenko: Analysis

Concerning **increasing the effort** of perpetrators, existing security failed to make Litvinenko a *hardened target*, despite an earlier attempt to poison him at the offices of a security company. Using liquid polonium-210 evidently required large-scale preparation and organisation. No routine attempts to *control weapons* could deter this plot without intelligence that an attack was imminent (which was evidently lacking).

Increasing the risks to the perpetrator includes enhancing *natural* and *formal surveillance*. There was no indication of a threat to Litvinenko at the hotel that could have suggested surveillance and might have led to prevention. Indeed, nothing noticeably untoward happened at the hotel meeting.

Turning to **reducing rewards** to the perpetrator British authorities sought to *deny benefits* by ensuring that Litvinenko's killers did not remain anonymous. Given that using polonium-210 indicated substantial resources and planning, an enquiry implicated Russia, despite their denials.

Turning to **reducing provocations** through *discouraging imitation* British authorities revealed outlines of the Litvinenko plot without details that would encourage its repetition. Showing that perpetrators could be identified was also intended to discourage future attacks.

Concerning **removing excuses** British authorities appointed an enquiry pointing to the use of polonium-210 and the implication that a major organisation, likely the Russian authorities, was responsible.

Georgi Markov

Markov: The Poisoning

Georgi Markov was born in 1929 near Sophia, Bulgaria. His father was an army officer, then worked in business. After university, Markov became a chemical engineer and a teacher before turning to writing. Some of his output, critical of communist Bulgaria, was banned (Lennon 2018). Visiting his brother in Italy in 1969, Markov requested a visa extension. When Bulgarian authorities refused, Markov defected to the West. Tried in Bulgaria in his absence he was sentenced to imprisonment as an enemy of the state (Volodarsky 2009).

Markov moved to London and in 1971 worked for the Bulgarian section of the BBC World Service. He continued criticising the Bulgarian regime including Zhivkov, the communist leader. Visiting Germany, he broadcast for CIA-funded Radio Free Europe (Emsley 2008, p. 3). In London, Markov spoke freely about the risks to his life (Hyams 2018). He married novelist Annabel Markova and the couple had a baby daughter.

On Wednesday, 7 September 1978, Markov was waiting for a commuter bus on the south end of Waterloo Bridge to take him to BBC Bush House for work. He later recalled feeling a stinging pain in his leg (BBC Radio 4 2018). Nearby, a man dropped an umbrella, retrieved it, then took a nearby taxi. Markov unsuspectingly continued to work.

On returning home to Balham about 10.30 pm Markov fell ill with vomiting and a fever. His wife telephoned a doctor, who suspected influenza. Annabel looked after her husband all night, and next day went to work leaving Georgi at home to recover. Later the doctor made a home visit and, finding Markov's condition considerably worse, summoned an ambulance (Emsley 2008, pp. 18–19).

Taken to St James's Hospital, Balham, Markov mentioned a mark on his leg, to house physician Bernard Riley. The medic arranged an X-ray, but it showed only an apparent blemish on the film. Markov's blood pressure was low, and his white blood cell count extremely elevated. On Saturday, 10 September, Markov was transferred to intensive care, but his condition continued to worsen. He died on Monday, 12 September.

In January 1979, an inquest reflecting autopsy findings judged that Markov had been 'unlawfully killed' by poisoning from a metallic pellet found in his thigh. Tests of both pellet and thigh tissue at the Chemical Defence establishment at Porton Down, Wiltshire, indicated ricin poison. The Police Forensic Science Laboratory established that the tiny pellet was engineered with two cavities with a combined volume of only 0.4 mg, suggesting that it held a substance lethal in minute amounts (Emsley 2008, pp. 14–15). Seemingly, Markov had been poisoned by a device (possibly an adapted umbrella or a gas or air pistol) introducing a pellet containing ricin into his leg (BBC Radio 4 2018).

At the time, the Bulgarian government claimed that the CIA had likely assassinated Markov, dispensing of his services at Radio Free Europe. However, after the regime collapse in 1989, newly available files pointed to the involvement of a Bulgarian secret service agent. One suspect was Francesco Gullino, a native Italian who became a Danish citizen. No charges have ever been brought.

Markov: Analysis

Concerning **increasing the effort** of perpetrators, Markov had criticised the Bulgarian regime, broadcast for CIA-funded radio, and recognised risks to his life, yet was not sufficiently a *hardened target* to escape assassination. Furthermore, domestic efforts to *control weapons* were evaded by using a disguised device possibly smuggled into the United Kingdom.

Among techniques to **increase the risk** to perpetrators, *assisting natural surveillance* was ineffective. Because of a disguised weapon, its use in a busy area, and the calculated delay in poisoning, potential witnesses and Markov himself were unalerted. This allowed the perpetrators to escape with no heightened risk.

Turning to **reducing rewards** to the perpetrator, in the Markov killing, the benefits to the Bulgarians included that Zhivkov was rid of an influential critic. Also, the assassination acted as a warning to other critics. Bulgarian authorities could deny involvement to evade diplomatic consequences because the perpetrators escaped. British authorities tried to *deny benefits* to the Bulgarian government by revealing part of the modus operandi and publicising likely Bulgarian involvement.

Turning to **reducing provocations**, the provocation from the Bulgarian standpoint was Markov's criticism of their regime and the British government's granting him asylum. British authorities sought to *discourage imitation* and deter similar attacks by publicising the assassination. But this risked revealing too much of the modus operandi, and showed that the assassination plot had been successful, hardly an outcome likely to discourage others.

SCP Overview

Increase Perpetrators' Effort

Regarding *hardening targets*, the Skripals were insufficiently protected. However, later, effective police and media warnings alerted the general public as secondary targets. Any security precautions surrounding Kim Jong-nam failed to avert his assassination. Seemingly, after setting up the attackers, the puppet masters escaped without attracting suspicion. Authorities remained unaware of an attempt to poison Litvinenko weeks before the successful assassination and of the sophisticated polonium plot. Markov had criticised the Bulgarian regime and knew the risk to his life, yet any safety precautions were circumnavigated. Overall, poison assassination plots evaded security arrangements and only secondary target hardening was effective where there was a public threat.

Controlling tools/weapons was ineffective where assassinations and attempts evaded domestic legal restrictions on poisons. It appears that smuggling into the United Kingdom enabled the use of Novichok against the Skripals, polonium against Litvinenko, and a disguised weapon and ricin against Markov. With Kim Jong-nam procedures to control weapons in Kuala Lumpur airport were seemingly skirted by using binary chemicals.

Increase Perpetrators' Risks

Following the Skripal attack, the public were alerted to use *natural surveillance* while authorities heightened *formal surveillance*. This helped protect the public from further contact with Novichok. But it was secondary protection after the attack, and the perpetrators escaped. In Kuala Lumpur airport, CCTV *formal surveillance* helped identify an attacker. Kim Jong-nam also reported the attack to airport staff. At the meeting between Litvinenko and other Russians in London, hotel *surveillance* could hardly have prevented the poisoning, because nothing noticeably untoward happened. In the Markov killing *natural surveillance* was ineffective. A disguised weapon, a busy area, and delayed action poisoning all rendered Markov and potential witnesses unaware, allowing the perpetrators to escape.

Reduce Perpetrators' Rewards

Turning to *concealing or removing targets* the Skripals were not concealed from would-be assassins. However, the rewards to the perpetrators were reduced by the Skripals' lives being saved, and they were later removed to a secret location. Kim Jong-nam was not sufficiently concealed from the attack in a public yet designated space where security precautions may have been considered less necessary.

The attackers were *denied the benefits* of a successful assassination because the Skripals survived, and Russian diplomats expelled. British authorities sought to prevent the perpetrators from disclaiming responsibility for killing Litvinenko by highlighting the resources required in using polonium-210 and holding an enquiry implicating Russia. Bulgarian authorities benefitted from Markov's assassination which eliminated an influential critic and warned other dissenters. They could officially deny involvement and evade consequences because the perpetrators escaped. British authorities responded by revealing the broad modus operandi and claiming likely Bulgarian involvement.

Reducing Provocations

A key approach is to *discourage imitation* of attacks, for example by publicity. Following Kim Jong-nam's assassination, Malaysian authorities published information about the modus operandi. With Litvinenko and Markov British authorities publicised information on the attacks and the identity of likely perpetrators. However, as these three plots were successful and those involved escaped, imitation was hardly discouraged. Regarding the Skripals, the international diplomatic reprisals aimed to discourage imitation and any future attempts.

Removing Excuses

With the Skripal attack, excuses denying Russian involvement were removed by investigations by police and Bellingcat, releasing CCTV footage, and unmasking the alleged attackers. The North Korean claim that Kim Jong-nam died of a heart attack was countered by toxicological evidence implicating nerve agent. In challenging excuses in the Litvinenko assassination, British authorities appointed an enquiry highlighting the use of polonium-210 and accusing Russian authorities. When the Bulgarian regime denied involvement in the Markov assassination, blaming the CIA, British authorities highlighted the plot's sophistication and implicated Bulgaria, a view later confirmed.

Means, Motive, Opportunity, Location, and Perpetrator-Victim Relationship.

Means

In the Skripal attack Novichok (A234) was applied to the door handle of their Salisbury home. While it allowed the assailants to escape, it was unreliable, risking others being poisoned while not guaranteeing the target being killed (as events proved).

In the killing of Kim Jong-un, it seems, each assailant applied to his face a binary chemical which combined to form VX, so protecting each perpetrator from the effects of the compound. If they were patsies, their escape did not need to be planned because if caught they would have no useful knowledge of the plot.

Administering slow-acting poison in tea allowed Litvinenko's killers to escape unsuspected. However, contamination caused by the poison enabled investigators to reconstruct events.

In the Markov assassination too, clandestinely injecting a ricin pellet and its delayed effect allowed assailants to get away. The secretive nature of the attack made it difficult to reconstruct events. The slow painful deaths of Litvinenko and Markov were a deterrent to other dissidents or defectors.

Motive

Litvinenko's attackers, one of whom knew him, likely had a personal element of motivation. However, with Kim Jong-nam, there could be no personal motive if the assailants were patsies. Regarding Skripal and Markov, no known personal connection existed between assailant and victim.

Various motives likely drove those who planned and directed the poisonings. The Skripal attack was presumably to revenge treason. Kim Jong-nam's assassination removed a critic of the North Korean regime. Litvinenko was killed for his defection and criticisms of the FSB. Markov's assassination removed a critic of the Bulgarian system. All the attacks aimed to deter others.

Opportunity

Opportunity to apply poison to the house door in Salisbury was guided by Sergei Skripal's routine, visiting the graves of his wife and son at the local cemetery on Sunday mornings. Plotters clearly knew Kim Jong-nam's travel and transit arrangements and exploited the busy airport to enable strangers to approach unchallenged.

A business relationship between Litvinenko and the main perpetrator allowed face-to-face contact to be arranged. The attacker's knowledge that Litvinenko was likely to drink tea enhanced their opportunity. Opportunity to kill Markov arose from the predictability of his journey to work, while the method of killing allowed the attack to go relatively unnoticed.

In all four instances, opportunity was created by the perpetrators using knowledge of the victims' routines and preferences to time the attack, or to aid the means of administering the poison.

Location

The location of Skripal's house for the poisoning assumes that the victims would encounter the treated areas and become contaminated. If contamination was minimal, this might explain why their illness manifested itself later in the centre of Salisbury, rather than immediately on contact with the poison.

Kuala Lumpur airport may have been chosen for the assassination of Kim Jong-nam because it allowed strangers to approach unchallenged. However, the presence of CCTV cameras, as events showed, ran the risk of perpetrators being identified.

In the Litvinenko killing, the hotel bar location facilitated the poisoning. It was entirely unsuspicious that drinks including tea should be ordered and consumed there.

The public location of the attack on Markov allowed his main assassin to escape. The positioning of the assassin(s), the taxi in which the umbrella carrier escaped, and the cover of other uninvolved people were all benefits of the location.

Perpetrator-Victim Relationship

Sergei Skripal, 66, was a well-educated, highly trained former colonel in the Russian GRU, enabling him to work for a long period as a double agent for the UK secret service. Yulia Skripal, 33, graduated from university, joined Nike in Russia, and later worked in the United Kingdom in business. Perpetrator Anatoly Chepiga, 39, graduated from military school, and following military service became a GRU colonel. His colleague Dr Alexander Mishkin, 39, trained as a physician for the Russian naval armed forces before joining the GRU. Victims and perpetrators were Russian. Sergei Skripal and the perpetrators had a military and intelligence background. These common features and political events brought them together.

Victim Kim Jong-nam, 45, was in line to lead North Korea. Politically exiled, his power was curtailed. One perpetrator Doan Thi Huong was a 28-year-old Vietnamese woman from a farming family. She worked in an entertainment outlet and did modelling (Foreign Staff, February 2017). The other perpetrator Siti Aisyah was a 25-year-old divorced Indonesian woman who worked in a Kuala Lumpur night club. The attackers were likely dupes. Indeed, in 2019, charges were dropped against Siti Aisyah, and Doan Thi Huong pleaded guilty to a lesser charge, leading to the release of both women. No prior relationship was evident between the victim and direct perpetrators which aided the escape of the organisers (Babulal 2017).

Victim Litvinenko was a 44-year-old former spy and Russian defector. Andrei Lugovoi, 40, was a former KGB officer who became a businessman. Dmitry Kovtun had grown up with him and had attended the Soviet Military Command Academy. Both victim and perpetrators had a shared language, country of birth, and background in intelligence. When Lugovoi was head of security at Berezovsky's television channel, Litvinenko had met him, providing a reason for them subsequently to meet for business. So, unlike the poisonings of Skripals, Kim Jong-nam, and Markov, face-to-face contact was justifiable.

Markov was born Bulgaria in 1929, the son of an army officer and later businessman. Following work as a chemical engineer and a teacher, he became a successful writer before defecting to the West. The main perpetrators were likely agents of the Bulgarian secret service, the main suspect being agent Francesco Gullino. At his death, Markov was 49 and Gullino was 32. Both suspected assailant and victim were Caucasian males of similar middle-class social backgrounds. Occupationally they occupied different political poles—dissident writer and secret service agent—and had no personal relationship.

Conclusion

Situational Crime Prevention and Assassination

Successful assassination plots, by design, circumvent security arrangements for the primary target, although secondary *target hardening* can be effective with a public threat. *Controlling* poison as a *weapon* tends not to deter assassination attacks despite domestic legal restrictions. Controls are circumvented by smuggling into the planned location the chemicals or poisons, and any equipment required.

Assassinations using poison are usually designed to avoid natural and formal *surveillance*, enabling the perpetrators to escape. The secretive nature of poisoning helps ensure that the victim and witnesses are unaware of any attack. Formal CCTV surveillance helps identify suspects but usually after their escape. Following an attack, authorities may encourage public vigilance if the poison has contaminated surroundings.

Potential assassination *targets can be protected (concealed)* and can take their own precautions, so successful perpetrators must discover their movements. Victims who survive can be moved to a safe location. Assassins and their operators are *denied benefits* of an attack if the victim(s) survive. Where the assassination succeeds, further perpetrator benefits can be denied by economic or diplomatic retaliation. Naming and shaming perpetrators removes the benefits of anonymity. However, being identified can aid perpetrators if the assassination is meant to deter critics of a regime.

Authorities at the receiving end of an attack may try to *discourage imitation* after the event by publicising outlines of the modus operandi, implying that future perpetrators will be caught. However, if the attackers have escaped, this defeats the purpose, and publicising too much detail risks encouraging future attacks.

Excuses often involve the organisers denying involvement in assassination and accusing others, made easier if perpetrators have escaped unobserved. Authorities at the receiving end *remove* such *excuses* by presenting evidence such as toxicology results, indications of state involvement, and information about alleged attackers.

Means, Motive, Opportunity, Location, and Perpetrator-Victim Relationship in Assassinations

As a *means* of killing a poison with delayed action can allow the perpetrator to escape. Slow poisoning gives no indication to potential witnesses of any attack so that even if traced, they are unlikely to recall anything pertinent. Also, where poisoning results in a long, painful death, it can deter others.

The background political *motive* for poisoning may be to exact revenge, to create a warning to others, or to remove a nuisance. *Opportunity* for carrying out the killing may take advantage of the victim's routines and preferences. *Location* is likely to be chosen to allow the attack to be carried out unnoticed or little noticed, and to enable the perpetrator to escape.

With political assassinations, the characteristics of *victim and perpetrator* may be similar if they were from military or intelligence backgrounds. Usually there is no direct personal relationship between perpetrator and victim, but where there is it can be used to the assassin's advantage.

Suggested Activities

Read the 19-page *CIA Manual* (c1954). Highlight the sections concerning the use of poison as a method of assassination.

Note examples of the wider use of poison in assassination from the examples given in the present chapter and from elsewhere. Consider how the latest technology can extend the use of poison for assassination, for example in ways that the poison is administered to the victim.

Key Text

Urban, M. (2018). *The Skripal Files: The Life and Near Death of a Russian Spy*. London: Macmillan.
A detailed look at a recent assassination attempt.

References

Anders, K. (1967). *Murder to Order*. New York, NY: The Devin-Adair Company.

Babulal, V. (2017, February 17). Jong-nam Murder: Indonesian Suspect 'Siti Aisha' Worked in KL Night Club Say Reports. *New Straits Times*. Retrieved from https://sg.news.yahoo.com/jong-nam-murder-indonesian-suspect-081608811.html.

BBC. (2018, October 8). Russian Spy Poisoning: What We Know So Far. Retrieved from www.bbc.co.uk/news/uk-43315636.

BBC News. (2019, March 11). Kim Jong-nam: Indonesian Woman Freed in Murder Case. *BBC News*. Retrieved from www.bbc.co.uk/news/world-asia-47520443.

BBC Radio 4. (2018). The Murder of Georgi Markov. *The Reunion*. Retrieved from www.bbc.co.uk/sounds/play/b0bgblcd. (Originally Broadcast 31 August 2018).

Bellingcat Investigation Team. (2018a, September 26). Skripal Suspect Boshirov Identified as GRU Colonel Anatoliy Chepiga. Retrieved from www.bellingcat.com/news/uk-and-europe/2018/09/26/skripal-suspect-boshirov-identified-gru-colonel-anatoliy-chepiga/.

Bellingcat Investigation Team. (2018b, October 9). Full Report: Skripal Poisoning Suspect Dr Alexander Mishkin Herpo of Russia. Retrieved from www.bellingcat.com/news/uk-and-europe/2018/10/09/full-report-skripal-poisoning-suspect-dr-alexander-mishkin-hero-russia/.

CIA Manual. (c1954). See Doyle, K. & Kornbluh, P. (Eds.). (2017). CIA and Assassinations: The Guatemala 1954 Documents. *National Security Archive Electronic Briefing Book No. 4* (Document 2 'A Study in Assassinations – Unsigned, Undated'). Retrieved from https://nsarchive2.gwu.edu/NSAEBB/NSAEBB4/.

Cobain, I., Vasagar, J., & Sample, I. (2006, December 8). Hotel Bar Staff Poisoned with Polonium 210. *The Guardian*. Retrieved from www.theguardian.com/uk/2006/dec/08/russia.topstories3.

Daily Excelsior. (2019, January 20). Kim Jong Nam Murder Trial Adjourned Again Until March. *DailyExcellsior.Com*. Retrieved from http://www.dailyexcelsior.com/kim-jong-nam-murder-trial-adjourned-again-until-march.

De Witte, L. ([1999]/2002). *The Assassination of Lumumba*. New York, NY: Verso (Translated from the Dutch by Ann Wright and Renée Fenby).

Dunkerley, W. (2016, February 5). Six Reasons You Can't Take the Litvinenko Report Seriously. *The Guardian*. Retrieved from www.theguardian.com/world/2016/feb/05/litvinenko-report-get-it-wrong-putin.

Emmott, R., & Balmforth, T. (2019, January 21). EU Sanctions Skripal Suspects – Russia Calls Move Groundless. *Reuters*.

Emsley, J. (2008). *Molecules of Murder*. London: Royal Society of Chemistry.

Escalante, F. (Commentary) (2008). *The Secret Assassination Report: CIA Targets Fidel* (With Commentary by the Former Head of Cuban State Security). London: Ocean Press.

Foreign Staff. (2017, February). Suspect in Kim Jong-un Assassination Posed in Flowery Bikini at Motor Show. *The Telegraph*. Retrieved from www.telegraph.co.uk/news/2017/02/24/suspect-kim-jong-nam-assassination.

Goldfarb, A., & Litvinenko, M. (2007). *Death of a Dissident: Alexander Litvinenko and the Return of the KGB*. (Free Press ed.). New York, NY: Simon and Schuster.

Harding, L. (2015, February 9). Litvinenko Told of Mysterious Break in at Mayfair Office. *The Guardian*. Retrieved from www.theguardian.com/world/2015/feb/09/litvinenko-inquiry-told-of-mysterious-break-in-at-mayfair-office.

Harley, N, & Sawer, P. (2018, March 11). Sergei Skripal Poisoning: Military Remove Ambulances and Police Cars for Nerve Agent Testing. *The Telegraph*. Retrieved from www.telegraph.co.uk/news/2018/03/10/spy-poisoning-military-remove-ambulances-police-cars-testing/.

Hyams, J. (2018, March 7). Georgi Markov: The Bulgarian Dissident Killed by a Poisoned Umbrella. *Express*. Retrieved from www.express.co.uk/life-style/life/928368/Georgi-Markov-Bulgarian-dissident-poisoned-umbrella.

Lee, A. S. (2003, June 23). Secret Lives. *Time*. Retrieved from www.time.com/time/magazine/article/0%2C9171%2C460254-1%2C00.html.

Lennon, T. (2018, September 10). Bulgarian Dissident Georgi Markov 'Shot' by Killer Poison Pellet from an Umbrella. *The Daily Telegraph*. Retrieved from www.dailytelegraph.com.au/news/bulgarian-dissident-georgi-markov-shot-by-killer-poison-pellet-from-an-umbrella/news-story/1263538e609b4927eb d103bc8f3ac3c2.

Litvinenko, A., & Felshstinsky, Y. (2007). *Blowing Up Russia: The Secret Plot to Bring Back KGB Terror*. New York, NY: Encounter Books.

Owen, Sir Robert. (2016, January). *The Litvinenko Inquiry: A Report into the Death of Alexander Litvinenko*. London: Her Majesty's Stationary Office. Retrieved from https://assets.publishing.service.gov.uk/government/uploads/system/uploads/attachment_data/file/493860/The-Litvinenko-Inquiry-H-C-695-web.pdf.

Reporter. (2016, January 20). Litvinenko Inquiry 'Theatre of the Absurd'. *The Irish Times*.

Sixsmith, M. (2007). *The Litvinenko File: The True Story of a Death Foretold*. London: Macmillan.

Tchouteu, J. (2017). *A Death in Geneva That Put a Nation in a Coma and Traumatised Africa: The Assassination of Félix-Roland Moumié and Cameroon's Unfinished Liberation*. New York, NY: Tisi Books.

Urban, M. (2018). *The Skripal Files: The Life and Near Death of a Russian Spy*. London: Macmillan.

Volodarsky, B. (2009). *The KGBs Poison Factory: Form Lenin to Litvinenko*. Minneapolis, MN: Zenith Press (Chapter 2).

Watts, J., & Branigan, T. (2012, January 17). North Korea's Leader Will Not Last Long Says Kim Jong-un's Brother. *The Guardian*. Retrieved from www.theguardian.com/world/2012/jan/17/north-korea-leader-not-long.

Wise, D., & Ross, T. B. (1967). *The Espionage Establishment*. New York, NY: Random House.

5

Terrorist Acts Using Poison

Introduction

I consider attempts to characterise and define terrorism. As a historical example of terrorist poisoning, I discuss the Nakam group plots to revenge Holocaust victims. More recently, terrorist poison plots and attacks in the United Kingdom have included those of Husnain Rashid convicted in 2018, and Kamel Bourgass sentenced in 2003. A 1994 sarin attack in the city of Matsumoto, Japan, was followed a year later by one on the Tokyo subway. In Chicago, in 1982, a perpetrator introduced potassium cyanide into drug capsules. I analyse these incidents using the framework of Situational Crime Prevention (SCP). Terrorism involving poison is also considered in relation to means, motive, opportunity, location, and perpetrator-victim relationships.

© The Author(s) 2020
M. Farrell, *Criminology of Poisoning Contexts*,
https://doi.org/10.1007/978-3-030-40830-5_5

What Is Terrorism?

Examples of terrorism spring to mind readily, from the 2001 attack on the New York twin towers, to the stabbings near London Bridge by Usman Khan in November 2019. Defining terrorism is difficult however and attempts have not attracted universal agreement.

General depictions refer to 'the use of violence … to achieve political aims or to force a government to do something' (www.collinsdictionary. com) or 'the systematic use of terror especially as a means of coercion' (www.merriam-webster.com). A US legal code defines terrorism as 'premeditated, politically motivated violence perpetrated against noncombatant targets by subnational groups or clandestine agent' (Legal Information Institute 2019).

Innes and Levi (2017) helpfully draw attention to three necessary conditions. Firstly, terrorism involves 'political violence' in that it is carried out in the pursuit of a 'political objective'. Next, terrorism is characterised by 'communicative violence', involving 'a desire to communicate an intimidatory message beyond the immediate victims'. Finally, terrorism implies an 'asymmetry of power' and arises when 'a relatively powerless group identifies a need to mobilise a response to a more powerful adversary'. Some commentators contest this last characteristic as it makes an unwarranted distinction between the terrorist acts of states and such acts perpetrated by citizens (ibid., p. 457). See also for example the Jamestown Foundation www.jamestown.org, a Washington, DC–based institute aiming to inform and educate policy makers about events and trends strategically important to the United States.

Terrorism Using Poison in Recent History—Nakam

Nakam (Hebrew for 'revenge') was a group of about 50 Holocaust survivors formed after the Second World War. Led by Abba Kovner, the group vowed to revenge Holocaust deaths by killing Nazis and Germans. Plans focused on Nuremberg as a former centre of Nazi activity.

In the first plot, the aim was to kill numerous Germans indiscriminately. Kovner visited Mandatory Palestine to obtain large quantities of poison to contaminate Nuremberg's water supply. Returning by sea via Toulon, France, Kovner became aware that he was suspected and ditched much of the poison overboard before being arrested by British authorities. Kovner spent two months in jail, after which he seemingly took no further part in Nakam.

In 1946, the group adopted another plan—to poison German prisoners of war held in Germany by US forces. Situated near Nuremberg was a bakery that supplied the Langwasser internment camp. Infiltrating both business and camp, members of the group poisoned thousands of loaves of bread with arsenic. Many prisoners became sick, but none died from poisoning (Porat [2000]/2009). Hoffman (2017) provides an overview of terrorism and 'irregular warfare' in a comprehensive text. Please also see Shea (2013, pp. 11–12) and Johnston (2017, passim).

Situational Crime Prevention Outline

Situational Crime Prevention links each of five general strategies with five opportunity-reducing techniques. Techniques to **increase the effort** of perpetrators are 'target harden', 'control access to facilities', 'screen exits', 'deflect offenders', and 'control tools/weapons'. **Increase the risks** concerns 'extend guardianship', 'assist natural surveillance', 'reduce anonymity', 'utilise place managers', and 'strengthen formal surveillance'. Techniques to **reduce rewards** to the perpetrator are 'conceal targets', 'remove targets', 'identify property', 'disrupt markets', and 'deny benefits'. Regarding **reduce provocations**, techniques comprise 'reduce frustrations and stress', 'avoid disputes', 'reduce emotional arousal', 'neutralise peer pressure', and 'discourage imitation'. **Remove excuses** concerns 'set rules', 'post instructions', 'alert conscience', 'assist compliance', and 'control drugs and alcohol'.

Terrorism and Situational Crime Prevention

In the following subsections, I am indebted to the research assessment on crime prevention and terrorism provided by Freilich et al. (2018). Clarke and Newman (2006) argue for applying SCP techniques to preventing terrorism, focusing on 'situated context' rather than only individual offender background. Terrorism tends to be ideological unlike other forms of crime to which SCP is applied. However, like other crimes it can involve motive, commitment and planning, peer networks, and exploiting opportunities. Accordingly, limiting opportunities for ideologically driven offenders to transgress could reduce terrorism. Clarke and Newman (2006) propose a 'four-pillar' opportunity structure of terrorist activities: selection of targets, choice of weapons, use of tools, and conditions facilitating terrorism.

Selection of Targets—EVIL DONE

Some critics suggest that terrorists can choose many potential targets, and it is impossible to protect all of them, thus limiting the application of SCP (e.g. Mueller 2010). However, Clarke and Newman (2006) maintain that some targets are more attractive to terrorists, and therefore represent higher risk needing greater protection. Their terrorism target risk assessment template with the acronym EVIL DONE indicates higher risk targets.

Exposed targets are especially visible and prominent (e.g. skyscrapers).
Vital targets provide essential functions (e.g. power plants).
Iconic targets have symbolic significance (e.g. government buildings).
Legitimate targets are considered deserving of attack (e.g. opponents' military installations).

Destructible targets are comparatively easy to eliminate.
Occupied targets are likely to contain many potential victims.
Nearer targets are closer to the terrorists and easier to travel to.
Easy targets have little security or are more accessible.

Considering these factors can help identify more likely targets allowing them to be prioritised for greater protection and situational interventions (see also, Newman 2009; Boba 2009).

Romyn and Kebbell (2018) identified the more important attributes of target selection as Occupied, Iconic, Easy, and Destructible. Other attributes—Exposed, Vital, and Near—were less important. Legitimate was too subjective (ibid., p. 591). Researchers recognise that ideology can influence target selection (Drake 1998). Typically, jihadists in the United States target Jews, homosexuals, and American society broadly. Far-right ideologists aim for government, police, and minorities (homosexuals, racial, ethnic, and religious groups). Extreme-left terrorists target corporations and animal testing laboratories. Ideology influences perceptions of potential targets, for example how an offender might interpret opportunities (Freilich and Chermak 2009). Accordingly, accounting for ideology situationally in the EVIL DONE template may make it more useful.

Weapons—MURDEROUS

Contending that certain weapons are attractive to terrorists, Clarke and Newman (2006) summarise their greater risk in the acronym MURDEROUS.

Multipurpose weapons are usable in various situations.
Undetectable weapons are concealed easily.
Removable weapons are easily handled and carried.
Destructive weapons cause maximum death and injury.
Enjoyable weapons are 'fun' to use.
Reliable weapons are expected to work smoothly.
Obtainable weapons are easily available for use.
Uncomplicated weapons are simple to use, requiring little training.
Safe weapons minimise the danger to the terrorist.

It follows that authorities can: evaluate how terrorists view these dimensions as aiding specific types of crimes, identify offenders' preferred weapons, and develop strategies to prevent their acquisition.

Tools

Terrorist tools (as well as weapons) include transportation used to gain access to targets and fake identification such as passports allowing them to travel freely without suspicion. Access to such tools increases the chances of successful terrorist attacks. Effective situational interventions aim to deny terrorists access to these tools, so changing the 'opportunity structure'.

Facilitating Conditions—ESEER

Facilitating conditions enabling terrorist acts relate to border security, banking security, immigration policy, and laws limiting access to weapons. While not directly implicated, these factors can have situational implications on terrorists' access to tools and weapons (Freilich and Chermak 2009). Facilitating conditions with examples are summarised in the acronym ESEER.

Easy conditions (a corrupt government or an organisation steeped in bribery)
Safe conditions (a country with loose requirements for identification)
Excusable conditions (government over-reactions that advantage terrorists)
Enticing conditions (communities that support terrorist actions)
Rewarding conditions (monetary or religious)

The approach recognises the many ways of anticipating how terrorists exploit opportunities. Consequently, it highlights crime-specific opportunities available for committing terrorism. Each form (e.g. suicide bombing, hijacking, or shooting) offers different opportunities and vulnerabilities on which terrorists capitalise. Once implemented the effectiveness of an intervention to tackle terrorism can be evaluated.

Husnain Rashid, UK

Rashid—The Case

Husnain Rashid, 34, of Nelson, Lancashire, England, worked at a local mosque. A supporter of the Islamic State, he was arrested in November 2017. Rashid was accused of providing internet information encouraging lone attackers. This included proposing attacks on the Trafford Centre shopping mall, Manchester, and inciting a plan to target young Prince George (an heir to the British throne). Poison plots included plans for contaminating supermarket ice-cream and injecting cyanide into groceries displayed in stores. Rashid was jailed in July 2018 after admitting several terrorist offences (Saddique and Halliday 2018).

Rashid made extensive attempts to conceal his on-line extremist propaganda from authorities. Intelligence agencies were unable to penetrate his laptop encryption. To publish on-line material, he used the encrypted messaging app 'Telegram' on three different SIM cards (small circuit boards). Among its features, Telegram offers Secret Chats where messages self-destruct once sent, making them accessible only to the intended user.

Rashid also hacked into a neighbour's internet connections. Most of his activity was conducted on a smartphone with no SIM card, on airplane mode (which disables the phone's wireless transmission functions), and with a tape over the camera. All this reflects counter-surveillance techniques.

In contrast to his sophisticated concealment was the Chaplinesque nature of Rashid's arrest. When officers arrived, he threw the smartphone out of the back door where it landed at the feet of a police officer.

Rashid—Analysis

Regarding **increasing the effort** of perpetrators, drugs and some food stuffs are in a sense *hardened* as *targets* by being packaged more safely. Technology like RFID (radiofrequency identification) tagging can also help. This uses small devices to track and identify items through a tag (a transponder), a reader (a scanning antennae and receiver), and an application system. However, the threat of someone poisoning accessible foods at Rashid's incitement would be difficult to prevent. *Screening exits* in stores typically involves the presence of security staff, general staff alertness, and merchandising security tags to prevent theft. But a terrorist might contaminate food in the store, or buy, poison, and discreetly return the consumables. This poses risks for the perpetrator in shops with security surveillance cameras but may be feasible in small stores without such surveillance.

Turning to **increasing the risks** to the perpetrator, once aware of Rashid's extraordinary steps to conceal his communications, intelligence agencies would have *strengthened formal surveillance.*

Concerning **reducing rewards** to the perpetrator *removing targets* applies to intelligence agencies protecting recipients of Rashid's propaganda (also *denying* Rashid the *benefit* of inciting them). Also, *removing targets* and *concealing targets* apply to proposed victims. Prince George's security could be enhanced. But any potential victims of poisoning store foods could not be removed or concealed because they are unspecified.

Turning to **reducing provocations**, *reducing emotional arousal* applies to controlling and intercepting Rashid's violence-inciting internet activity. *Discouraging imitation* relates to managing publicity. Authorities informed the media of some of Rashid's steps to avoid detection, but exact details of how intelligence agencies monitored his internet activity remained guarded.

Concerning **removing excuses** none of the techniques appears to be relevant.

Kamel Bourgass UK Ricin Plot

Bourgass—The Case

Information emerged from Algerian agencies through their questioning of a detainee Mohamed Meguerba, in Algeria. (Some journalists later intimated that torture was used to obtain the information.) Algerian sources alerted UK authorities to an address in North London and possible terrorist activity. Accordingly, in January 2003, anti-terrorist squad officers raided a flat in Wood Green, North London, and discovered a suspected chemical weapons laboratory.

Police found castor oil beans and fruit stones suspected of being kept to produce ricin and cyanide respectively. Recipes were found for making ricin, cyanide, botulism, and nicotine. Six suspects were arrested on the day of the raid and one other was detained two days later.

A further suspect Kamel Bourgass, who had been living in the flat, fled to Bournemouth on the south coast of England, from where he circuitously made his way to Manchester. Police launched a nationwide search for the suspected al-Qaeda operative. Nine days after the London raid, police tracked Bourgass to a flat in Manchester. During this raid he stabbed several police officers, killing one of them, Detective Constable Oake (Summers 2005). In June 2004, Bourgass was jailed for the murder (BBC 13 April 2005).

In 2005, Bourgass was tried for conspiracy to cause a public nuisance by using poisons and or explosives to create disruption, fear, or injury. Police stated that he had planned to spread ricin-based paste on handrails in the London underground and on buses.

Prosecuting counsel Nigel Sweeney QC stated that Bourgass and nine other men, all North Africans, were involved in a conspiracy between January 2002 and the time of their arrest.

Bourgass claimed that he had written the poison recipes for Meguerba (the informant) to help him to kill bandits in his village in Algeria. Bourgass was sentenced to 17 years in jail for the conspiracy (BBC 13 April 2005). Remaining suspects were released without charge, had their trials abandoned, or were acquitted (Summers 2005). (Please also see Shea and Gottron 2013, passim.)

Bourgass—Analysis

Increasing the effort of perpetrators by *controlling weapons* applies to the poisons Bourgass proposed to use. The terrorists tried to circumvent legal controls by developing homemade toxins, but police thwarted this.

Turning to **increasing the risks** to perpetrators, *assisting natural sur-veillance* includes supporting whistle blowers. With Bourgass, informa-tion precipitating the raid on the Wood Green flat apparently came from an Algerian detainee, possibly but not certainly through voluntary whis-tle blowing. *Strengthening formal surveillance* applied to the police and anti-terrorist scrutiny leading to police raids.

The ability to **reduce rewards** to the perpetrator was limited because Bourgass's plot was to use poison in public places, making it difficult for authorities to forewarn people except generally. Also, where an attack or even a thwarted plot is publicised, terrorists may see the fear generated among citizens as a reward.

Turning to **reducing provocations**, authorities tried to *discourage imi-tation* or copycat crimes, for example by not releasing the poison recipes.

Bourgass's claim that he wrote poison recipes for Meguerba to combat gangs in Algeria was an **excuse removed** by the evidence of poison manu-facture in the London flat.

The Matsumoto and Tokyo Terrorist Attacks 1994 and 1995

The Matsumoto Attack

On 27 June 1994, members of the Aum Shinrikyo doomsday cult in Japan perpetrated a gas attack in the city of Matsumoto. It aimed to kill three judges and to test the lethal capacity of sarin nerve agent. The target was the dormitory apartments of the judges whom the cult expected to find against them in an upcoming lawsuit. Aum Shinrikyo members parked an adapted refrigerator truck nearby containing liquid sarin (secretly manufactured by the cult). At around 10.40 pm, a heating device in the vehicle converted the fluid into gas. A fan dispersed this towards the apartment building (Olson 1999).

Soon, paramedics were ferrying to hospital multiple casualties suffer-ing symptoms including eye problems, nausea, and headaches. People who were near open windows or in air-conditioned rooms were exposed to the lethal gas. Five residents were discovered dead in their homes and two died soon after arriving at hospital. An eighth victim Sumito Kono (whose innocent husband was initially suspected of the killings) became comatose from the gas and died in 2008 (Reporter, 6 August 2008). All three judges were affected but not fatally. About 200 people were treated in hospital, staying at least overnight (Olson 1999).

Police received an anonymous tip implicating Aum Shinrikyo after the Matsumoto attack. However, the cult was not officially implicated until after the Tokyo subway murders eight months later (Olson 1999).

The Tokyo Subway Attack

On 20 March 1995 Aum Shinrikyo followers released sarin into the Tokyo subway. Twelve people were killed, and another died later from the poison. An estimated 5500 were injured (Pletcher 2019).

Five men entered the subway system on the morning of 20 March. Each joined different subway lines converging on central Tokyo's Tsukiji station. At around 8 am each attacker dropped sealed bags of sarin on their carriage floor and punctured the bag with a sharpened umbrella tip. They then left the train station and drove away in a waiting car. Meanwhile, in each train the deadly liquid vaporised and affected passengers as the vehicle continued into the city centre. Passengers left the carriages at each stop where their clothing contaminated others and fumes spread. Two subway staff died after trying to remove punctured sarin bags at Kasumigaseki station (Pletcher 2019). Asahara Shoko, the cult leader, may have known that police planned a March raid on AUM premises and launched the subway attack to preoccupy them.

Two days after the attack, police had identified AUM as the organiser. They raided AUM offices in Tokyo and the group's laboratory in Kamikuishiki, Yamanashi prefecture, seizing toxic chemicals used to manufacture sarin. In May 1994 police arrested Shoko and other principal members. It was July 2018 before Shoko and six senior cult members were executed (Pletcher 2019). Please see also Kaplan (1995) and Murakami ([1997, 1998]/2003).

The Matsumoto and the Tokyo Poisonings—Analysis

Regarding **increasing the effort** to the perpetrator, the Matsumoto attack was not officially linked to Aum Shinrikyo despite a reported tipoff. In the Tokyo attack, authorities could not effectively *control access to facilities* or *screen exits* because neither transport staff nor police knew of the impending threat. Any attempt to *control tools/weapons* was evaded as perpetrators manufactured their own poison and dispersed it clandestinely.

Turning to **increasing the risks** to perpetrators, *natural* and *formal surveillance* might have deterred the Matsumoto attack. Targets were specific (the three judges) and Aum Shinrikyo's antipathy to them was discoverable. Prior intelligence might have alerted police, although whistle blowing would be deterred by the cult's secretiveness. Following the Matsumoto incident, it is uncertain whether better *natural and formal surveillance* could have revealed the Tokyo plot. In Tokyo the victims were random, and not directly linked to cult members. At best, authorities might have had a general awareness of the possibility of a sarin attack on public transport.

Reducing rewards to the perpetrator includes *removing targets*. In the Matsumoto attack, the cult's secretiveness denied authorities advance intelligence. For the Tokyo subway murders, the transport authorities and first responders strove to get passengers off the system. But staff who died after touching suspect containers were unaware of the need for protective clothing and equipment.

Turning to **reduce provocations**, in neither attack was it possible to *neutralise peer pressure*. Any pre-emptive attempts at disruption were forestalled by the cult's secrecy.

Similarly, **removing excuses** did not apply. AUM recognised the harm they would cause and needed no 'excuses' for the murders, convinced they were acting for a higher cause (see also Clarke 2009).

Chicago Tylenol Tampering

Chicago Tylenol Tampering—The Case

In a Chicago suburb on the morning of 29 September 1982, Mary Kellerman, aged 12, woke and complained of having a cold. Her parents gave her pain killers. A few hours later, Mary was dead. Later the same morning in another part of the city, Adam Janus, a postal worker, suddenly died. His brother and sister-in-law, grieving over Adam's death and suffering headaches, took pain relief medication. They also died. Over a two-day period, seven people lost their lives. Linking these incidents was that all the deceased had taken an over-the-counter painkiller, Extra Strength Tylenol (acetaminophen) (Fletcher 2009).

It emerged that these capsules were laced with potassium cyanide. The pills came from different production plants. They had been sold in different Chicago drug stores—downtown, Arlington Heights, Grove Village, Schaumberg, and Winfield (Emsley 2008, p. 173). Police concluded that the medication had been tampered with at the various points of sale, possibly by someone buying or stealing the product, adding poison, then returning it secretly to the store shelves.

Having linked the Chicago deaths, police used loudspeakers to warn residents against taking Tylenol. Stores stripped the product from their shelves. Manufacturer Johnson and Johnson promptly recalled their products from stores, warned the public of the risks including through a media campaign, and offered to replace purchased capsules with tablet equivalents free of charge (Rehak 2002).

In the longer term, federal laws were framed against tampering and improvements were made to the packaging of over-the-counter products to make it tamper proof and tamper responsive. Furthermore, the manufacturing process was made more secure. No suspect was charged or convicted of the Tylenol poisonings. In October 1982 James William Lewis, a New York tax consultant, attempted to blackmail Johnson and Johnson and claimed responsibility for the deaths, but later denied this. Convicted of extortion, he spent 12 years in jail. As well as the seven people killed in the original poisoning, others died in later copycat crimes.

Chicago Tylenol Tampering—Analysis

Regarding **increasing the effort** of perpetrators, efforts to *harden targets* concerned both Tylenol and intended victims. Johnson and Johnson recalled the capsules and offered free replacements, while retailers cleared their shelves. More widely, safer packaging was developed for drugs and foods. Concerning potential targets of further poisoning, police warned Chicago residents. Crucially, it was recognised that police alone could not stop such crimes. They needed help from others with the competence and facilities to implement necessary prevention techniques. Accordingly, police, federal agencies, local authorities, private corporations, retail outlets, and manufacturing sources worked together to tackle the problem.

Concerning **increasing the risks** to perpetrators, *extending guardianship* applies to the police linking Tylenol with the Chicago deaths. Later copycat crimes were combatted by *assisting natural surveillance* of shoppers and *strengthening formal surveillance* by storekeepers and local police. Also, media outlets warned people about copycat product tampering.

Turning to **reducing rewards**, by providing information and warnings to Chicago residents, police *removed potential targets* of the perpetrator. Similarly, media and police later alerted the public to the risk of copycat tampering.

With reference to **reducing provocation**, techniques included *discouraging imitation*. Although copycat crimes followed the Tylenol killings, they were likely minimised by safer packaging and better security during manufacture.

Techniques for **removing excuses** of the perpetrators appear not to apply.

Outsmarting Terrorists Overview

Selection of Targets—EVIL DONE

Recall that Clarke and Newman (2006) identified targets at increased terrorist risk, as being Exposed, Vital, Iconic, Legitimate, Destructible,

Occupied, Nearer, and Easy. In Husnain Rashid's plots involving food stores, proposed targets were *occupied, near, and easy* to access. Bourgass's plot was to poison areas of the London underground and buses representing *vital, occupied, near, and easy* to access targets. In the Matsumoto attack the judges' dormitory apartments were *near* but otherwise posed difficulties for using dispersed gas, making the attempt unsuccessful. The Tokyo subway (Pletcher 2019) was *vital* for public transport, *occupied* by many passengers, *near* for terrorists to reach, and *easy* to access. In the Tylenol poisonings (Fletcher 2009) the shops and the drugs they sold were *easy* to access and presumably *near* in that any such shop could be targeted.

Weapons—MURDEROUS

Clarke and Newman (2006) warn against the terrorist use of weapons that are Multipurpose, Undetectable, Removable, Destructive, Enjoyable, Reliable, Obtainable, Uncomplicated, and Safe. Prevention involves evaluating how terrorists view these dimensions as aiding specific types of crimes; identifying the weapons terrorists most seek; and developing strategies to prevent access to them. While the proposed use of poison envisaged by Rashid could have been *destructive* and affected many people, it would not have been *undetectable*. Similarly, Bourgass's plot could have been highly *destructive*. In the Matsumoto attack, the poison was *destructive* but not *reliable* (the intended targets—the judges—were not killed). In the Tokyo subway attack (Pletcher 2019) sarin proved to be *destructive*, comparatively *reliable*, and relatively *safe* for the trained perpetrators. The Chicago Tylenol poison (Fletcher 2009) was *destructive* and *reliable* but not *undetectable*.

Tools

A notable instance of financing tools for terrorism is the Aum Shinrikyo sarin attacks. In Matsumoto perpetrators used a converted truck to generate poison gas. For the Tokyo attack the poison was prepared in the cult's secret factories.

Facilitating Conditions—ESEER

Clarke and Newman (2006) summarise factors acting as facilitating conditions to terrorism as Easy, Safe, Excusable, Enticing, and Rewarding. The crimes of Rashid, Bourgass, and Aum Shinrikyo seemed enabled by the *enticing conditions* of a subculture justifying and encouraging attacks against a perceived hostile society. For some, there was the *rewarding condition* of an anticipated religious salvation.

Overview of SCP and Terrorism

Increase the Effort of Perpetrators

Against Rashid's incitements to poison loose store groceries, prevention might involve *hardening targets* by packaging them all. Following the Tylenol poisonings, authorities hardened targets by modifying product packaging and warning Chicago residents of the danger.

Regarding *controlling access to facilities* authorities did not improve their control of access to the Tokyo subway, being unaware of the impending threat. Today, authorities better recognise that transport systems can attract terrorism and that they require greater protection (Clarke and Newman 2006).

Relating to Rashid's plot, *screening exits* in stores typically involves preventing theft. This is circumvented by a perpetrator poisoning food in situ, or removing it, contaminating it, and replacing it. In the Tokyo killings, authorities did not focus on screening exits, being unaware of the threat.

Bourgass planned to evade legal *controls on tools/weapons* by producing homemade poisons but police thwarted this. In the Tokyo poisonings, perpetrators used their own manufactured supply.

Increase the Risks to Perpetrators

In the Tylenol tampering police *extended guardianship* by investigating and identifying the common link between the Chicago deaths.

By *strengthening formal surveillance*, authorities detected Rashid's terrorist communications. Preventers strive to keep ahead as terrorists continually adapt to avoid detection. Indeed, authorities scrutinise how their own techniques and technology can be circumvented and keep adapting accordingly. *Assisting natural surveillance* relating to a detainee may have aided Bourgass's arrest. In the Matsumoto and Tokyo attacks any surveillance was avoided by Aum Shinrikyo's secrecy and the lack of connection between the Tokyo targets and cult members. Following the Tylenol poisonings, copycat crimes were countered by *natural* and *formal surveillance* involving shoppers, storekeepers, and local police, aided by media outlets.

Reduce Rewards to the Perpetrator

In monitoring recipients of Rashid's propaganda, intelligence agencies *removed* them as *targets*. Transport staff and first responders helped get passengers off the Tokyo subway. In the Chicago Tylenol attacks products were recalled from stores and residents were warned.

Because of the action of authorities, Rashid was *denied benefits* of inciting followers of his propaganda.

Reduce Provocations

Intelligence services *reduced the emotional arousal* of others who might have been incited to violence by intercepting Rashid's internet communications.

In the Matsumoto and Tokyo attacks, Aum Shinrikyo's secrecy prevented authorities from *neutralising peer pressure* to disrupt their plans.

Authorities *discouraged imitation* by limiting information on Rashid's modus operandi and details of counter-intelligence activity. Similarly, authorities withheld exact details of Bourgass's plot. Copycat crimes after the Chicago Tylenol attacks were minimised by introducing legislation and improving packaging and manufacturing safety.

Remove Excuses

Terrorism's ideological nature blunts techniques aimed at removing excuses. AUM needed no excuses for their attacks, being convinced that they were acting justly. Bourgass's excuse that he wrote poison recipes to help Meguerba combat gangs in Algeria was shaken by the discovery of a domestic poison factory.

Means, Motive, Opportunity, Location, and Perpetrator-Victim Relationships.

Means

Rashid incited others to poison food in stores. Bourgass's flat contained equipment, ingredients, and recipes to make ricin, cyanide, botulism, and nicotine. Sarin was dispersed from a truck in the Matsumoto attack and released from bags in the Tokyo poisoning Cyanide was introduced into Tylenol capsules in stores. Importantly, both Rashid and Bourgass plotted to leave poisons (in stores, on the public transport system) and escape. Indeed, the Tylenol poisoner was never caught. The Matsumoto attackers escaped in their adapted truck, and the Tokyo perpetrators walked safely away. All this allowed the killing to occur when the perpetrator was elsewhere, leaving victims unaware of the danger.

Motive

Motives for terrorist attacks tend to be ideological so that targets are broad groups or random victims. Rashid incited others to poison 'infidels' in the community. Bourgass proposed to poison members of society in public places. Exceptionally, in Matsumoto Aum Shinrikyo intended to poison judges considered antipathetic, but inadvertently killed other residents, making it seem a random terrorist killing. In the Tokyo attack random passengers and transport staff were killed. Although the perpetrator(s) of the Tylenol poisonings were not caught the motive was likely to kill indiscriminately.

Opportunity

Opportunity to perpetrate terrorist attacks arises from their comparative unpredictability. Important work highlighting more vulnerable types of targets like the EVIL DONE template (Clarke and Newman 2006) points to increased risks. However, precise indications of proposed targets require direct intelligence. Rashid incited others to exploit the comparatively unsupervised access to store groceries. Bourgass planned to contaminate public places in London which might be less supervised. The Matsumoto gassing was time constrained by the imminent court case against Aum Shinrikyo, leading to a planned but flawed attack. In the Tokyo attack terrorists targeted the transport network at a busy time when the release of sarin would attract least attention. Whoever perpetrated the Tylenol poisonings exploited the then-existing opportunity to tamper with over-the-counter drugs.

Location

Rashid incited targeting stores where easy access allowed tampering with goods. Similarly, the Tylenol poisonings capitalised on stores selling medication. Bourgass planned to contaminate public transport. In Matsumoto a truck parked on a public road released gas towards an apartment block. The Tokyo attack targeted the busy public transport network. In these instances, the proposed or actual location was accessible and freely used by the public, allowing perpetrators scope for their crimes.

Perpetrator-Victim Relationship

In terrorist attacks targeting the general public, perpetrator and victim are rarely directly connected. Exceptionally, one aim of the Matsumoto attack was to kill the three judges in a legal sense 'connected' with cult members.

Husnain Rashid, 34, of Nelson, Lancashire, England, lived at home with his parents and taught at a local mosque. His technology skills enabled him to set up systems to avoid detection in his terrorist communications. A fanatical supporter of the Islamic State, his proposed victims were 'infidels'.

Kamel Bourgass (one of many aliases) was an Algerian illegal immigrant in his early 30s, who came to the United Kingdom in 2000 using the name Nadir Habra. His proposed victims were members of society in general. Indeed, the judge in his case referred his aim to 'destabilise society' (Campbell et al. 2005).

Perpetrators of the Matsumoto and Tokyo attacks were members of the cult Aum Shinrikyo led by Asahara Shoko (Pletcher 2019). Among the main perpetrators of the Tokyo attack was physician Ikuo Hayashi. Graduating from Keio University he worked as a heart specialist at Keio Hospital and later at the National Sanitorium Hospital, north of Tokyo. In 1990 he joined AUM. Following the subway attack and having helped police investigations, Hayashi was sentenced to life imprisonment. Other perpetrators included Kenichi Hirose, 30, who gained a postgraduate degree in physics at Waseda University. Toru Toyoda, 27, held a degree in applied physics from the University of Tokyo. Both Hirose and Toyoda joined AUM's chemical brigade. Masato Yokoyama, 39, graduated in applied physics at Tokai University and then worked for an electronics firm. He became AUM's undersecretary at their Ministry of Science and Technology. Yasuo Hayashi, 37, graduated in artificial intelligence at Kogakuin University. He joined AUM's Ministry of Science and Technology. After sentencing and appeals, Shoko, Hirose, Toyoda, Yokoyama, and Hayashi were hanged in July 2018 (Reporter 2018).

In the Tokyo subway poisonings 12 people died directly from the sarin and one person died years later having been comatose from the effects. As well as passengers, two staff died from contamination after trying to assist at Kasumigaseki station (Pletcher 2019) including Kazumasa Takahashi, 50, an assistant stationmaster (Kitazawa 2019). Around a thousand people were non-fatally injured. There was no relationship between perpetrators and victims.

In the Chicago Tylenol poisoning the perpetrator is unknown. Victims were Mary Kellerman a 12-year-old schoolgirl; Adam Janus, 27, a postal worker; Stanley Janus, 25 (Adam's brother); and Theresa Janus, 19 (Stanley's wife). Four other Chicago residents were also poisoned (Fletcher 2009). Even after the product's recall, there were further victims: Mary Reiner, 27, of Winfield Illinois; Paula Prince, 35, a stewardess with United Airlines, found dead in her Chicago apartment; and Mary McFarland, 35, of Elmhurst, Illinois (Emsley 2008, pp. 173–174). Any connection between the unknown perpetrator and victims is unlikely, given the randomness of people purchasing and taking the contaminated drug.

Conclusion

Targets, Weapons, Tools, and Facilitating Conditions

Vulnerable targets are Exposed, Vital, Iconic, Legitimate, Destructible, Occupied, Nearer, and Easy. In the Tylenol poisoning, stores presumably were *near* and *easy* to access. In Rashid's plots involving food stores, proposed targets were *occupied, near, and easy* to access. Bourgass's plot involving London transport represented *vital, occupied, near, and easy* to access targets. In the Matsumoto attack the judges' dormitory apartments were *near* but otherwise posed difficulties thwarting the attempt. Tokyo subway was *vital, occupied, near* for terrorists, and *easy* to access. Prevention involves using specific intelligence, better protecting higher risk targets, and continuing awareness of variations of attacks such as product tampering.

Terrorists choose weapons that are Multipurpose, Undetectable, Removable, Destructive, Enjoyable, Reliable, Obtainable, Uncomplicated, and Safe. Terrorist poisoning tends to be *destructive* and comparatively *safe* for perpetrators, but not *undetectable*. Its use can be unreliable as in Matsumoto or comparatively *reliable* as with the Tokyo attack.

Tools used in the Aum Shinrikyo attacks included disguised transport generating poison gas, and poison manufactured in AUM factories.

Facilitating conditions make attacks Easy, Safe, Excusable, Enticing, Rewarding. For some terrorists, a subculture offers *enticing conditions* justifying and encouraging attacks against society. The *rewarding condition* of a presumed religious salvation may contribute.

SCP and Terrorism

Terrorism thrives on unpredictability, increasing the fear it inspires. Identified *targets can be hardened*. Foods or drugs can be protected by safer packaging and authorities can warn intended victims. *Access to facilities can be controlled* and *exits screened* by higher staffing and better security. But protecting busy stores, public spaces, and public transport is challenging. Although poisons as *weapons are controlled*, terrorists can make their own.

Police and others can *extend guardianship* by finding a common link between deaths. Predicting attacks is problematic where there is no seeming relationship between victims and terrorists. However, certain types of targets can be identified as posing greater risk allowing security to be improved, and sometimes potential perpetrators to be identified.

Strengthening formal surveillance includes monitoring suspects' communication and its concealment. *Assisting natural surveillance* includes supporting whistle blowers, but the secretiveness of terrorist organisations inhibits this. *Natural* and *formal surveillance* can be more effective after a terrorist incident when similar attacks are expected.

Removing targets can involve intelligence agencies preventing material inciting violence or hatred from reaching proposed targets; rescuing people targeted in attacks; and removing substances intended to harm others. Terrorists are *denied benefits* of inciting followers where propaganda is blocked.

Authorities can *reduce emotional arousal* by intercepting violence-inciting terrorist internet activity. Authorities' attempts to *neutralise peer pressure* among terrorists and their supporters are hindered by the secretiveness of terrorist organisations. Authorities try to *discourage imitation* of offences by withholding crucial details, by legislation and heavy sentencing, and by tightening security gaps that allowed the original offence.

With ideologically driven terrorist groups, techniques to *remove excuses* are limited because perpetrators make no excuses, convinced they are justified. Terrorists' false justifications may be countered by hard evidence. A pre-emptive approach to combat radicalisation especially through the internet is challenging.

Means, Motive, Opportunity, Location, and Perpetrator-Victim Relationship

Using poison in terrorist attacks facilitates a perpetrator's escape. Both Rashid and Bourgass intended to leave poisons and get away, and the Tylenol poisoner was never caught. In Matsumoto, attackers escaped in their truck, and in Tokyo they walked to waiting cars. Poisons can kill when the perpetrator is elsewhere, leaving victims unaware of the danger.

Victims of ideological terrorism tend to be groups or random people rather than specifically targeted individuals. Where terrorists despise their host culture, their diffuse motive may be to harm 'society'.

Opportunity for terrorist attacks arises from comparatively free access to stores, public places, and transport networks and is tackled by identifying higher risk targets or using specific intelligence.

Terrorist attacks using poison tend towards accessible and freely used locations allowing perpetrators to introduce poison and ensure the public are affected.

Terrorists usually have no personal connection with their victims who are generally people going about their daily business. In organised terrorist groups, members may be highly educated, with specialist knowledge and skills, and deployed accordingly.

Suggested Activities

Identify a recent example of terrorism using poison and review it relative to: targets, weapons, tools, and facilitating conditions; techniques of situational prevention; and means, motive, opportunity, location, and perpetrator-victim relationships.

What are the findings of each approach and how do they differ and correspond?

Compare your findings to those extrapolated from the case examined for the present chapter. What are the similarities and differences and the reasons for them?

Key Texts

Freilich, J. D., & Newman, G. R. (Eds.). (2009). *Reducing Terrorism Through Situational Crime Prevention*. Crime Prevention Studies, Vol. 25. Boulder, CO: Lynne Rienner Publishers.

This comprises several chapters each examining aspects of applying SCP to terrorism.

Hoffman, B. (2017). *Inside Terrorism: Columbia Studies in Terrorism and Irregular Warfare* (3rd ed.). New York, NY: Columbia University Press.

This book concerns the historical evolution of terrorism and terrorist mentality. It analyses developments in global terrorism—adversaries, motivations, strategies, and tactics. The author considers the likelihood of a chemical, biological, radiological, or nuclear terrorist strikes.

References

BBC. (2005, April 13). Killer Jailed Over Poison Plot. *BBC News*. Retrieved from http://news.bbc.co.uk/1/hi/uk/4433709.stm.

Boba, R. 'Evil Done' (2009) in Freilich, J. D., & Newman, G. R. (Eds.) *Reducing Terrorism Through Situational Crime Prevention*. Crime Prevention Studies, Vol. 25. Boulder, CO: Lynne Rienner Publishers (pp. 71–91).

Campbell, D., Dodd, V., Norton-Taylor, R., & Cowan, R. (2005, April 14, Thursday). Police Killer Get 17 Years for Poison Plot. *The Guardian*.

Clarke, W. R. (2009). Bioterrorism: A SCP Approach. In J. D. Freilich & G. R. Newman (Eds.), *Reducing Terrorism Through Situational Crime Prevention* (pp. 93–109). Crime prevention studies, Vol. 25. Boulder, CO: Lynne Rienner Publishers.

Clarke, R. V. G., & Newman, G. R. (2006). *Outsmarting the Terrorists*. Westport, CT: ABC-CLIO.

Drake, C. J. M. (1998). The Role of Ideology in Terrorists' Target Selection. *Terrorism and Political Violence, 10*, 53–85.

Emsley, J. (2008). *Molecules of Murder: Criminal Molecules and Classic Cases*. Cambridge: The Royal Society of Chemistry (RSC Publishing).

Fletcher, D. (2009, February 9). A Brief History of the Tylenol Poisonings. *Time*. Retrieved from http://content.time.com/time/nation/article/0,8599,1878063,00.html.

Freilich, J. D. and Chermak, S. M. (2009) 'Preventing Deadly Encounters Between Law Enforcement and American Far-Rightists' in Freilich, J. D., and Newman, G. R. (Eds.). (2009) *Reducing Terrorism Through Situational Crime Prevention*. Crime Prevention Studies, Vol. 25. Boulder, CO: Lynne Rienner Publishers. (pp. 141–172).

Freilich, J. D., Gruenewald, J., & Mandala, M. (2018, October). Situational Crime Prevention and Terrorism: An Assessment of Ten Years of Research. *Criminal Justice Policy Review*, 1–29. Retrieved from https://www.researchgate.net/publication/328257967SituationalCrimePreventionandTerrorismAnAssessmentof10YearsofResearch.

Hoffman, B. (2017). *Inside Terrorism: Columbia Studies in Terrorism and Irregular Warfare* (3rd ed.). New York, NY: Columbia University Press.

Innes, M., & Levi, M. (2017). Making and Managing Terrorism and Counter-Terrorism: The View from Criminology. In A. Liebling, S. Maruna, & L. McAra (Eds.), *The Oxford Handbook of Criminology* (6th ed., pp. 455–477). Oxford: Oxford University Press. (Chapter 20,.

Johnston, W. R. (Compiler) (2017, December 5). *Chemical Attacks in War and in Terrorist Attacks*. Retrieved from http://www.johnstonsarchive.net/terrorism/chembioattacks.html.

Kaplan, D. E. (1995). Aum Shinrikyo. In Tucker, J. B. (Ed.). (2000). *Toxic Terror: Assessing Terrorist Use of Chemical and Biological Weapons*. Cambridge, MA: MIT Press.

Kitazawa, T. (2019, March 20). Kin, Station Staff Hold Memorial for Victims of '95 Sarin Gas Attack. *The Asahi Shimbun*. Retrieved from http://www.asahi.com/ajw/articles/AJ201903200059.html.

Legal Information Institute. (2019). Title 22 Chapter 38 US Code Section 2656f *Annual Country Reports on Terrorism*. Retrieved from https://www.law.cornell.edu/uscode/text/22/2656f.

Mueller, J. (2010). Assessing Measures Designed to Protect the Homeland. *Policy Studies Journal, 38*, 1–21.

Murakami, H. (2003 [1997, 1998]). *Underground: The Tokyo Gas Attack and the Japanese Psyche*. Vintage (Translated from the Japanese by Alfred Birnbaum and Philip Gabriel).

Newman, G. R. (2009). Reducing Terrorist Opportunities: A Framework for Foreign Policy. In J. D. Freilich & G. R. Newman (Eds.), *Reducing Terrorism Through Situational Crime Prevention* (pp. 33–59). Crime Prevention Studies, Vol. 25. Boulder, CO: Lynne Rienner Publishers.

Olson, K. B. (1999). Aum Shinrikyo: Once and Future Threat? *Bioterrorism* 5, 4, August 1999 (Centers for Disease Control and Prevention). Retrieved from https://wwwnc.cdc.gov/eid/article/5/4/99-0409_article.

Pletcher, K. (2019). Tokyo Subways Attack of 1995. *Encyclopaedia Britannica*. Retrieved from www.britannica.com/event/Tokyo-subway-attack-of-1995.

Porat, D. (2009 [2000]). *The Fall of the Sparrow: The Life and Times of Abba Kovner*. Palo Alto: Stanford University Press.

Rehak, J. (2002, March 23). Tylenol Made a Hero of Johnson & Johnson: The Recall That Started Them All. *New York Times*. Retrieved from www.nytimes.com/2002/03/23/your-money/IHT-tylenol-made-a-hero-of-johnson-johnson-the-recall-that-started.html.

Reporter. (2008, August 6). Survivor of Aum's '94 Sarin Attack Died While in Coma. *The Asahi Shimbun*. Retrieved from https://web.archive.org/web/20080919101928/http://www.asahi.com/english/Herald-asahi/TKY200808050477.html.

Reporter. (2018, July 26). Japan Hangs All 6 Remaining Aum Death Row Inmates. *Japan Times*.

Romyn, D., & Kebbell, M. R. (2018). Mock Terrorists Decisions' Concerning Use of the Internet for Target Selection: A Red-Team Approach. *Psychology, Crime and Law, 24*, 589–602.

Saddique, H., & Halliday, H. (2018, May 31). Isis Supporter Admits to Prince George School Attack Plot. *The Guardian*. Retrieved from https://www.the-guardian.com/uk-news/2018/may/31/isis-supporter-admits-to-prince-george-school-attack-plot-husnain-rashid.

Shea, D. A. (2013). *Chemical Weapons: A Summary Report of Characteristics and Effects.* Congressional Research Service 13 September 2013. Retrieved from https://fas.org/sgp/crs/nuke/R42862.pdf.

Shea, D. A., & Gottron, F. (2013). *Ricin: Background and Potential Role in Terrorism.* Congressional Research Service 17 April, 2013.

Summers, C. (2005, April 13). Questions Over Ricin Conspiracy. *BBC News.* Retrieved from http://news.bbc.co.uk/1/hi/uk/4433499.stm.

6

Poisoning in Warfare

Introduction

After defining warfare, I touch on examples of chemical agents, protection against them, and attempts to limit their use. Historical examples are discussed. The chapter then considers chemical attacks in Syria and Iraq. Regarding Syria, the chapter considers attacks on Khan Sheikhoun in 2017, Khanal-Assal in 2013, and Ghouta also in 2013. I also discuss the 1988 attack on the Kurdish city of Halabja, Northern Iraq. These conflicts are examined through Situational Crime Prevention and means, motive, opportunity, and location, as well as perpetrator–victim relationships.

Defining Warfare

General definitions of warfare refer to conflict and to 'the weapons and methods that are used' (Cambridge University Press 2019). Elaborating on this, Dupuy and Dupuy (2007 [1991]) describe the beginnings of warfare as primitive 'clashes of force'. The early combatants were 'groups of Palaeolithic men'. They were 'armed with crude stone implements' and

© The Author(s) 2020
M. Farrell, *Criminology of Poisoning Contexts*,
https://doi.org/10.1007/978-3-030-40830-5_6

fought over 'food, women or land' (Ibid., p. 1). Through history, the nature of the contesting groups, the weapons they use, and what they fight about have differed. Further features that can refine a definition are location, tactics, duration, and scale.

War may be between nations or groups of nations but may involve groups within a state as in civil war. Among weapons used since the days of 'crude stone implements' have been edge weapons such as swords and bayonets; projectiles such as arrows, spears, and catapult shot; guns ranging from handheld to huge fixed weapons; grenades, bombs, torpedoes, and rockets carrying warheads; and biological, chemical, and nuclear weapons. Reasons for fighting have included a desire to dominate and a wish for independence. War on land, sea, and air may soon be extended to space while location is a distinctive feature, for example in jungle and desert warfare. Tactics are reflected in the terms such as 'guerrilla warfare' and 'trench warfare'. War is usually lengthy and on a large scale.

Chemical Agents, Protection, and Attempts to Curtail the Use of Chemical Weapons

Groups of chemical agents used in warfare include nerve agents (VX, sarin), blister agents (sulphur mustard), choking agents (chlorine, phosgene), and blood agents (hydrogen cyanide). These are more fully described in Chap. 1.

Protection against chemical agents tends to be physical, although there are examples of medical interventions against them. Physical items such as gas masks and protective clothing limit exposure by protecting the eyes, lungs, and skin from chemical contact. Gas masks with chemical filters, such as activated charcoal, are effective against inhaled chemical agents. A protective garment guards against chemical weapons that cause harm upon skin contact. Military battle dress overgarments are generally cloth, containing a layer of charcoal-impregnated foam. Wearing both a mask and a suit provides full protection against most chemical exposures (Shea 2013, p. 8).

In 1997, the Chemical Weapons Convention treaty came into force, which prohibited developing, producing, stockpiling, transferring, and using chemical weapons and their precursors. Based in The Hague, the relevant administrative body is the Organisation for the Prohibition of Chemical Weapons (OPCW). Under the treaty, limited production is allowed, for example, for protective or medical purposes. Where chemical weapons are destroyed, it must be verified by the OPCW.

Historical Use of Chemical Weapons

First World War Use of Chemical Weapons

Although poisons have long been deployed in military conflict, it was the First World War that heralded modern chemical warfare. Both sides used chemical weapons including the choking agents chlorine and phosgene, the blister agent sulphur mustard, and, ineffectively, the blood agent hydrogen cyanide. An estimated million casualties were affected by chemical agents during the Great War (Ellison 2007, pp. 567–570).

The first largescale deployment occurred during April and May 1915 in the second battle of Ypres, Belgium, when German forces used chlorine gas (Thomas 2014, p. 9). Chlorine forms a greenish cloud and its effects can be reduced by covering the mouth with a wet cloth. Phosgene was developed to be deadlier and harder to detect (being colourless). However, its effects were delayed, allowing effected troops to continue immediate fighting which limited its impact. German forces used phosgene mixed with chlorine on British troops at Wieltje near Ypres on 19 December 1915, causing 69 deaths and over a thousand casualties (Edmonds 1993 [1932]).

Sulphur mustard was widely used during the First World War. Delivered in artillery shells, it settles in the ground as an oily liquid. Germany deployed it in July 1917 prior to the Third Battle of Ypres. British forces used it in September 1918 during the breaking of the Hindenburg line, a German defensive position on the Western Front (Heller 1984).

Reportedly, the United States and Italy tried hydrogen cyanide gas in 1918 but found that being lighter than air it quickly dispersed into the atmosphere, weakening its effectiveness (Schneditz 2008, p. 13).

Chemical Weapons in the Italo-Ethiopian War 1935–1936

In October 1935, following an Italian rigged border demarcation dispute between Ethiopia (Abyssinia) and Italian Somaliland, Italian forces entered Ethiopian territory beginning the Second Italo-Ethiopian War. General De Bono commanded the Italian forces, while Emperor Haile Selassie led the Ethiopians. Protecting their supply routes and attack lines, Italy deployed chemical weapons, mainly mustard gas, aiming to demoralise Ethiopian troops, disrupt communications, and confuse troop movements (Grip and Hart 2009, p. 3).

In December 1935 in the Takkaze Valley, Ethiopia, Italian aircraft dropped grenades of tear gas and asphyxiating gas. Initially sulphur mustard air bombs were released but later the Italians used aerial spray tanks. In 1936, Italy used chemical weapons at the Battle of Shire and elsewhere. In April that year, the Ethiopian government issued a list of towns said to have been attacked with chemical weapons (League of Nations, Letter 1936).

Chemical weapons led to a 'significant number' of deaths, although accurate figures are disputed (Grip and Hart 2009, p. 3; Stepanov and Popov 1962). Subsequently, Italy officially acknowledged its use of chemical weapons in Ethiopia, largely confirming previous allegations (Del Boca 1969).

Sino-Japanese War and the Battle of Changde 1943

Prior to and during the Second World War, Japan allegedly used chemical weapons against China, killing 10,000 people and injuring 80,000. Following the war, chemical agents left behind by the Japanese were found in China including pots containing sulphur mustard, phosgene, and lewisite—a vesicant and lung irritant (Notman 2014).

During the Second Sino-Japanese War, in 1943, a battle was fought at Changde, Hunan Province. The Japanese aimed to stretch the Chinese National Revolutionary Army, weakening their local strength and ability to reinforce the Burma campaign. Japanese forces used chemical weapons extensively in the engagement.

Situational Crime Prevention

Situational Crime Prevention (SCP) is fully described in the chapter 'Theory and Poison Contexts'. Briefly, five general strategies are each associated with five opportunity-reducing techniques. Regarding the strategy to **increase the effort** of perpetrators are the techniques 'target harden', 'control access to facilities', 'screen exits', 'deflect offenders', and 'control tools/weapons'. **Increase the risks** concerns 'extend guardianship', 'assist natural surveillance', 'reduce anonymity', 'utilise place managers', and 'strengthen formal surveillance'. For **reduce rewards** to the perpetrator, the techniques are 'conceal targets', 'remove targets', 'identify property', 'disrupt markets', and 'deny benefits'. **Reduce provocations** involves 'reduce frustrations and stress', 'avoid disputes', 'reduce emotional arousal', 'neutralise peer pressure', and 'discourage imitation'. **Remove excuses** concerns 'set rules', 'post instructions', 'alert conscience', 'assist compliance', and 'control drugs and alcohol'.

Syria and the Use of Chemical Weapons

The Syrian Civil War

From 2011, increasing protests against the Syrian government and calls to depose President Assad were suppressed, and violence escalated into armed conflict. The civil war involves the Ba'athist Syrian Arab Republic (led by Assad) coupled with domestic and foreign allies fighting domestic and foreign forces opposing the Syrian government (and one another) in different groupings. Factions include the Syrian government and armed forces and their allies; majority Sunni opposition rebel groups including the Free Syrian Army; the majority Kurdish Syrian Democratic Forces; Salafi (Sunni) Jihadists such as the al-Nusra Front; and the Islamic State of Iraq and the Levant (ISIL).

The Syrian Arab Republic and its forces are supported by Iran, Russia, and Hezbollah (the Lebanon-based Shi'a Islamist group). The Democratic Federation of Northern Syria and related Syrian Democratic Forces have US support. A 2014 US-led coalition conducted air strikes against ISIL and government and pro-government targets. Turkey, opposing the Syrian government, occupied areas of North Western Syria. Israel directed air strikes against Iranian forces and Hezbollah, opposing their presence in south-western Syria. Reported chemical attacks include those on Khan Sheikhoun in April 2017, Khanal-Assal in March 2013, and Ghouta in August 2013.

Khan Sheikhoun, Syria, April 2017—The Attack

A chemical attack attributed to Assad's forces was directed at the town of Khan Sheikhoun in the Idlib Province of north-western Syria in the morning (06:30 to 06:45 am) of 4 April 2017. At the time, Idib Province was largely controlled by 'rebel fighters' and jihadists linked to al-Qaeda (the militant Sunni Islamist organisation founded by Osama bin Laden) (BBC, April 2017).

Idlib Province health directorate, run by the opposition, claimed that at least 89 people were killed and 541 more injured. According to an April 2017 OPCW statement, analysis of autopsy samples from three victims indicated exposure to sarin or similar (BBC, 26 April 2017).

On Thursday 6 April, US president Trump ordered the firing of toma-hawk missiles on the Shayrat airbase suspected of launching the Khan Sheikhoun attack (Rosenfeld 2017). President Assad later denied using chemical weapons, accusing the West of fabricating the story as a pretext for the missile attack. Russian sources said that the Syrian air force had struck the eastern outskirts of Khan Sheikhoun in the late morning of 4 April 2017, but the target was a terrorist ammunition depot with work-shops producing chemical warfare munitions.

A document seemingly based on declassified French intelligence states that sarin was identified in samples collected from Khan Sheikhoun. Evidence was also found of the presence of hexamine (a stabiliser in sarin production) and diisopropyl methyl phosphonate, a by-product (National Evaluation, April 2017).

Khan Sheikhoun, Syria, April 2017—Analysis

SCP strategies to **increase the effort** of perpetrators include *controlling tools/weapons*, which can apply to reducing or preventing the future use of chemical weapons. The Chemical Weapons Convention and its related inspections attempts to exert such control. Acceding to the convention in September 2013, Syria agreed to destroy its chemical arsenal. In the Khan Sheikhoun attack, none of these controls was effective. Possibly, being in a civil war, the perpetrators avoided the pressure that could be exerted on waring countries for using chemical agents. Confusion about weapon access and territory enabled Russia to claim that the attack was on a terrorist source of chemical weapons. Another technique, *target hardening*, can involve minimising the impact of poison on the intended population. Gas masks and special protective clothing can be deployed for troops and civilians, and training given on how to use them. In Khan Sheikhoun, there was no such protection.

Increasing the risks to perpetrators includes 'assisting natural surveillance' and 'strengthening formal surveillance'. Surveillance includes witness reports of chemical weapons use, satellite images, and personal phone camera recordings. Following the **Khan Sheikhoun** attack, autopsy reports and environment samples indicated the presence of chemicals associated with sarin production (National Evaluation, April 2017). Surveillance can discourage further attacks where perpetrators realise that their actions will be revealed and they can be held responsible.

Among strategies that **reduce rewards** to the perpetrator are *concealing* people intended as *targets* of bombing raids. This depends on intelligence of where the bombing may take place and seems not to have arisen in the Khan Sheikhoun attack.

Turning to **reduce provocations**, within a war zone, *avoiding disputes* implies agreeing to safe zones for certain groups or designating separate areas for those fighting. In Khan Sheikhoun, there were no such arrangements. *Reducing emotional arousal* can apply to softening the rhetoric of leaders of the waring countries or areas. International pressure can de-escalate conflicts and a forum to discuss differences can help, but with Khan Sheikhoun international views were ineffectual.

In wartime, **remove excuses** relates to *setting rules* through internationally agreed conventions and challenging perpetrators who offer excuses for infringing these agreements. Accordingly, President Assad denied using chemical weapons and accused the United States of fabricating the story to justify their own missile attack. Russian sources accepted that the Syrian air force had struck the eastern outskirts of Khan Sheikhoun on 4 April 2017 but stated that the target was a terrorist ammunition depot with chemical agents. These statements were challenged via conventions disallowing chemical weapons. It was also claimed that sarin was identified in samples from Khan Sheikhoun, and that a stabiliser and a by-product of sarin production had been found (National Evaluation, April 2017).

Khanal-Assal, Aleppo, 19 March 2013—The Attack

During the Syrian civil war, in February and early March 2013, conflict involved the village of Khanal-Assal, 12 kilometres from Aleppo. Rebel forces shelled the village for several weeks and by 3 March controlled a Police Academy near the village, having killed the last of the government forces defending it. By mid-March, government forces held Khanal-Assal and the Syrian Army base nearby.

On 19 March 2013, between 7 and 7.30 am a rocket hit an area of houses and farmland releasing sarin gas. A wind carried the gas to a nearby neighbourhood where witnesses reported seeing some people convulsing or lying unconscious. At least 20 people reportedly died and over a hundred were injured (United Nations, 12 December 2013). Those affected were evacuated by local people and Syrian Army personnel to the University Hospital in Aleppo and other local hospitals. According to the

Syrian Observatory for Human Rights, the attack killed at least 26 people including government soldiers and civilians (Barnard 2013).

Both the Syrian government and opposition accused each other of the attack, but neither offered convincing documentation (BBC News, 19 March 2013a). While the Syrian government invited the United Nations to investigate the incident, disputes over investigational scope delayed matters. Meantime, the Syrian government asked Russia to send specialists to investigate, and site samples were collected indicating that sarin was used in the attack (Reuters, 9 July 2013). As the United States blamed the Syrian government, Russia held the opposition responsible. United Nations investigators arrived in Syria in August 2013 as larger-scale attacks took place against Ghouta on 21 August. It was December 2013 before the UN report was completed, finding that chemical weapons had likely been used in Khan al-Assal, and citing organophosphate poisoning (United Nations, 12 December 2013).

Khanal-Assal, Aleppo, 19 March 2013—Analysis

Among strategies to **increase the effort** of perpetrators *controlling tools/ weapons* by invoking international agreements and carrying out inspections did not prevent chemical weapons being used in Khanal-Assal. *Hardening targets* by minimising the impact of poison through wearing protections was not available to civilians, forces personnel, or even first responders (United Nations, 12 December 2013).

Among strategies to **increase the risks**, *assisting natural surveillance*, and *strengthening formal surveillance* can discourage future attacks where perpetrators believe that their actions will be revealed and that they will be held accountable. In the Khanal-Assal attack, disputes between the Syrian government and the United Nations about the remit of proposed investigations caused delays. A prompter investigation by Russian specialists found site evidence of sarin use (Reuters, 9 July 2013). But then Russia and the United States disagreed about who was responsible. Also, when UN investigators arrived in Syria in August 2013, the subsequent attacks on Ghouta may have de-prioritised the Khan al-Assal investigation.

To **reduce rewards** to the perpetrator, *concealing targets* can work with planned bombing raids but depends on accurate intelligence about the proposed location. In Khanal-Assal, chance prevailing winds influenced where the chemicals settled, limiting pre-emptive action by victims.

Turning to **reducing provocations**, *avoiding disputes* by agreeing safe zones, or separate areas for groups in conflict, did not arise regarding Khanal-Assal. Potential to *reduce emotional arousal* following the attack evaporated as the United States and Russia disputed culpability.

Removing excuses can involve *setting rules* by citing internationally agreed conventions and providing evidence of breaches. This might have helped counter any excuses in other circumstances, but events may have been overshadowed by the Ghouta attack.

Ghouta, Damascus, August 2013—The Attack

Eastern and Western Ghouta are suburbs of Damascus which in August 2013 were controlled by the Syrian opposition. Attacks were made on these suburbs on the morning of 21 August 2013. The first attack was on Eastern Ghouta at about 2.30 am. The area was a rebel weapons supply route from Jordan which had been under attack by Syrian forces and Hezbollah for several months (Hubbard et al. 2013). At least eight improvised rockets, carrying a chemical warhead, hit an area in the Zamalka and Ein Tarma neighbourhoods. Two laboratories subsequently examined samples from these areas. One or both laboratories found at least traces of sarin in 14 of 17 cases (Sellstrom et al. 2013). A second attack occurred in western Ghouta at about 5 am on 21 August but subsequently no chemical warheads were found, and environmental samples did not indicate the presence of sarin.

Public intelligence assessments from the United Kingdom and the United States said that the Syrian government used a nerve agent against opposition forces in Ghouta on 21 August 2013. Preliminary US estimates were of 1429 deaths (Office of the Press Secretary, the White House 2013). UK intelligence sources estimated 'at least 350 fatalities' (Chairman of the Joint Intelligence Committee, Joint Intelligence Organisation 2013). Other estimates were also in the hundreds (Human Rights Watch 2013).

Inspectors from a UN mission requested access to the Ghouta sites on 22 August to which three days later the Syrian Ba'athist government agreed. Inspectors visited Moadamiyah (western Ghouta) on 26 August and Zamalka and Ein Tarma (eastern Ghouta) on 28 and 29 August.

Members of the Arab League and the United States blamed Syrian forces for the attack. After a Paris meeting with league members, on 8 September 2013, Secretary of State John Kerry stated, 'All of us agree…that Assad's deplorable use of chemical weapons…crosses an international global red line' (Dickinson 2013). Russian president Putin argued that evidence was lacking that Syria had used chemical weapons (BBC, 27 August 2013b).

A UN Human Rights Council report the following year stated that 'Chemical weapons, specifically sarin, were found to have been used in multiple incidents during the conflict'. However, the report stated that, 'In no incident was the commission's evidentiary threshold met with respect to the perpetrator' (United Nations General Assembly Human Rights Council 2014, p. 2 summary).

Ghouta, Damascus, August 2013—Analysis

Regarding **increasing the effort** of perpetrators, *controlling tools/weapons* through chemical weapons agreements and inspections did not deter the Ghouta attack. Neither was there *target hardening* by providing troops and civilians with protective items.

Of strategies to **increase the risks**, *assist natural surveillance* and *strengthen formal surveillance* may deter further attacks where perpetrators believe they will be accountable. Following the Ghouta attacks, in the Zamalka and Ein Tarma neighbourhoods there was evidence of rockets carrying a chemical warhead and sarin traces (Sellstom et al. 2013). The Syrian government granted UN inspectors permission to visit the Ghouta sites within three days.

Among strategies that **reduce rewards** to the perpetrator *concealing targets* is possible with planned bombing raids given specific intelligence but was unavailable in the Ghouta attacks.

Turning to **reducing provocations**, *avoiding disputes* through agreeing safe zones or separate areas for groups in conflict was absent in Ghouta. There was the potential to *reduce emotional arousal* following the attack as UN inspectors were allowed into the area and environmental samples were gathered. However, this elicited contradictory claims from different parties. Arab League members and the United States blamed Syrian forces (Dickinson 2013), while Putin denied there being evidence of Syria using chemical weapons (BBC 27 August 2013b).

Concerning **remove excuses**, *setting rules* by citing conventions and showing breaches to counter excuses did not prevent the Ghouta attacks.

Iran-Iraq War and the attack on Halabja, Iraq 1988

Iran-Iraq War

The Iran-Iraq war extended from 1980 to 1988, preceded by increased territorial and political disputes. Iran was a very predominantly Shi'a state led by a revolutionary cleric Ayatollah Ruhollah Khomeini. Iraq also with a predominantly Shi'a population was led by President Saddam Hussein, whose rule was secular but who was born a Sunni. Hussein gave positions of power mainly to Sunni Arabs constituting only a fifth of the country's population.

Saddam Hussein disputed parts of the historical Iran-Iraq border. Iraq wanted control over Khuzestan, an oil-rich area in southwest Iran bordering Iraq. Hussein also feared the designs of Iran's revolutionary government to stir unrest among Iraq's majority Shi'ite population.

In September 1980, following claims that Iran had shelled Iraqi border posts, Iraqi forces invaded Western Iran on the joint border. They advanced into Khuzestan but failed to take the oil refining centre at Abadan. By December 1980, Iran was managing to hold back Iraqi forces about 50 miles (80 km) inside Iran. The following year and in 1982 Iran pushed back Iraqi forces, and Iraq withdrew its military from all occupied Iranian ground and sought peace.

Iran's leader the Shi'a cleric Ayatollah Khomeini continued the war hoping to overthrow President Hussein. There was stalemate.

In the middle of all this, long-running conflicts between Iraqis and Kurds reignited. Kurdish parties resisted Saddam Hussein, and the militias of the Kurdish Democratic Party and the Patriotic Union of Kurdistan were gaining military support from Iran. In 1986, Iraq strengthened a campaign to defeat Kurdish fighters in North Iraq and to attack the Kurdish population. Eventually, in 1988 a ceasefire was agreed between Iran and Iraq followed two years later by a formal peace agreement.

Attack on Halabja, Iraq

In 1988, with the Iran-Iraq war ending, an attack was launched on the Kurdish city of Halabja, Northern Iraq. Halabja is 150 miles north-east of the Iraqi capital Baghdad and 10 miles from the Iranian border. The action was part of the sustained Iraqi offensive against Kurds, and an attempt to combat an Iranian action aiming to capture the city of Sulaymaniyah—part of operation Zafar.

Following the occupation of Halabja by Iranian forces, the chemical attack was launched on the morning of 16 March 1988 (Organisation for the Prohibition of Chemical Weapons 2006). A UN medical investigation reported that mustard gas and unidentified nerve agents were used in the attack (Hiltermann 2007, p. 195). Iraqi jets were said to have swooped over Halabja for five hours spraying mustard gas and nerve agents possibly sarin, tabun, and VX (BBC News, 25 January 2010).

More recent assessments (de Bretton-Gordon 2016) speak of the pre-bombardment of the city to break windows and doors and to drive people to seek underground shelter before the air attack using mustard agent and sarin nerve agent. Being heavier than air and being in an area with exposed widows and door spaces, the chemicals could seep underground and into cellars and air-raid shelters. (The method foreshadowed the Ghouta attack many years later.)

The US Defence Intelligence Agency initially considered Iran responsible for the attack. Reports from the city indicated that Saddam Hussein's forces launched the chemical offensive. Further indications were that it was an Iraqi assault on Iranian forces, pro-Iranian Kurdish forces, and the citizens of Halabja (BBC On This Day, 16 March 1988). Hussein's deputy Ali Hassan al-Majid who ordered the attack on Halabja was tried for crimes against humanity towards the Kurds and executed in 2010 (Blomfield 2010).

Estimates of the numbers killed range from 3200 to 5000 with many more injured. One report is that 'about 5,000 people' died in the attack (BBC News, 25 January 2010). Many of the wounded were taken to hospitals in Tehran, the Iranian capital (BBC On This Day, 16 March 1988).

Attack on Halabja—Analysis

Concerning **increasing the effort** of perpetrators, *controlling tools/weapons* through chemical weapons agreements and inspections did not prevent the Halabja attack. Attempts were made to *harden targets* as Halabja residents hid from bombardment in underground refuges. However, this was exploited in an air attack with heavier-than-air poison gas (de Bretton-Gordon 2016).

Turning to **increasing the risks to perpetrators**, *assisting natural surveillance* and *strengthening formal surveillance* can include witness reports, satellite images, and recordings. Following the Halabja attack, a UN medical investigation reported that mustard gas and nerve agents were used (Hiltermann 2007, p. 195). Accountability and deterrence characterised the trial and execution of Ali Hassan al-Majid (Blomfield 2010).

Reducing rewards to the perpetrator by *concealing targets* failed in Halabja. This was because victims were duped by a pre-attack into taking underground cover before the subsequent chemical attack.

Regarding **reducing provocations**, in Halabja, there was no tactic of *avoiding disputes* by providing safe zones or separate areas for groups in conflict. Nor was there evidence of rival leaders' rhetoric being softened to *reduce emotional arousal*.

Concerning **removing excuses**, *setting rules* by invoking conventions to challenge excuses led ultimately to a charge of crimes against humanity and al-Majid's execution (Blomfield 2010).

Situational Crime Prevention Overview

We now consider the attacks in Syria and in Halabja, Iraq, together in relation to SCP.

Increasing the Effort of Perpetrators

Controlling tools/weapons through international chemical weapon agreements and inspections did not deter the attacks in Khan Sheikhoun, Khanal-Assal, and Ghouta. Embedded in a civil war, the conflicts were less amenable to control. Fluctuating territorial boundaries and confusion about access to weapons enabled Russian sources to variously deny any Syrian government involvement and claim that the attack was on a terrorist source of chemical weapons. While civil war may hinder correct attribution and deterrence, even in the Halabja attack, where state actors were involved, none of these controls worked.

Hardening targets through wearing protective items coupled with training for people likely to be targeted was not evident in Khan Sheikhoun, Ghouta, or Khanal-Assal, where even first responders were affected (United Nations, 12 December 2013). In Halabja, residents were attacked with poison gas after seeking protection in underground shelters (de Bretton-Gordon 2016).

Increase Risks to Perpetrators

Key techniques are enhancing *natural* and *formal surveillance*. Following the Khan Sheikhoun attack, autopsy evidence and environmental samples indicated chemicals associated with sarin production (National Evaluation, April 2017). In the Khanal-Assal attack, after disputes about UN investigations, Russian specialists found site evidence of sarin use, but Russia and the United States disagreed about culpability (Reuters, 9 July 2013). After Ghouta, observers found rockets carrying a chemical warhead and detected sarin traces in environment samples (Sellstom et al.

2013). Following the Halabja attack, a UN medical investigation reported that mustard gas and nerve agents were used (Hiltermann 2007, p. 195). Ali Hassan al-Majid's execution raised the hope that it might deter others.

Reduce Rewards

Reliable intelligence can enable victims as *targets* to be *concealed* but was absent in the Khan Sheikhoun and the Ghouta attacks. In Khanal-Assal, chance prevailing winds influenced where the chemicals settled, limiting pre-emptive action. In Halabja, victims were gassed after taking underground cover.

Reduce Provocations

Neither safe zones nor separate areas for warring groups were arranged to *avoid disputes* in Khan Sheikhoun, Khanal-Assal, Ghouta, or Halabja.

To *reduce emotional arousal* implies softening war rhetoric, exerting international pressure to de-escalate the conflict, and providing a negotiation forum. None of this deterred the attacks on Khan Sheikhoun or Halabja. Potential to de-escalate when outside entities investigated the Khanal-Assal attack evaporated amid arguments about attribution. Following the Ghouta attack, the United States and Russia, respectively, blamed and defended Syria (Dickinson 2013; BBC 27 August 2013b).

Remove Excuses

In wartime, *setting rules* can involve citing codes of conduct and evidence of transgression, so challenging perpetrator's excuses. Accordingly, Assad denied using chemical weapons on Khan Sheikhoun, while Russian sources claimed that the Syrian air force mistakenly hit that target while aiming for a terrorist ammunition depot. In response, implying the importance of international 'rules', evidence of sarin was identified in samples from Khan Sheikhoun (National Evaluation, April 2017). In

Halabja, the 'rules' informing crimes against humanity eventually led to al-Majid's execution (Blomfield 2010). With the Ghouta attack, the convention proved toothless.

Means, Motive, Opportunity, and Location, and Perpetrator–Victim Relationship

Means

In Khan Sheikhoun, the means of killing was an air attack using sarin or similar substances (National Evaluation, April 2017). In Khanal-Assal, sarin gas was released following a rocket impact (United Nations, 12 December 2013). In Ghouta, rockets carried a chemical warhead delivering sarin nerve agent. Halabja, Northern Iraq, was attacked by Iraqi jets spraying mustard gas and nerve agents possibly sarin, tabun, and VX (BBC News, 25 January 2010).

Where chemical weapons are used in war, it attracts abhorrence reflected in specific conventions and related inspection regimes aiming to abolish their use. This may reflect the power of chemical weapons to inspire terror. Such poisons can cause lingering death affecting the morale of surviving troops and terrifying civilians. Some chemicals such as colourless and odourless poisonous agents are hard to detect, making precautions difficult to implement.

Motive

In the Khan Sheikhoun attack, the motive of the Assad forces was to defeat or weaken the control of the rebel fighters and jihadists controlling the Idib Province (BBC, April 2017). Regarding Khanal-Assal, if the Syrian government were culpable, they wanted to deplete opposition forces and demoralise civilians when, in fact, they inadvertently killed members of their own forces. If opposition forces were responsible, they wanted to kill government forces (Hubbard et al. 2013). A spokesman for the Free Syrian Army accused the government of attacking its own people to smear the opposition (TIME 2013). In the Iraqi attack on Halabja, the motive was to deplete Iranian forces aiming to capture the city of Sulaymaniyah and to kill pro-Iranian Kurdish forces and the citizens of Halabja.

Opportunity

In the Khan Sheikhoun attack, opportunity was provided through minimising the risk to Syrian air forces by carrying out an early morning raid. In the event, a price was paid for the attack when President Trump ordered the launch of tomahawk missiles on the airbase reportedly used to launch the Khan Sheikhoun attack (Rosenfeld 2017). Regarding Khanal-Assal, the Syrian government (or opposition) seized the opportunity of the comparatively low risk of mounting a rocket attack. In Ghouta, risk to attackers was reduced by carrying out a night-time rocket offensive. In Halabja, Northern Iraq, there was opportunity to carry out a low-risk attack by using aircraft to spray chemical agents and to simultaneously harm Iranian forces, Kurds, and civilians. The Iraqi forces took the opportunity to inflict maximum harm by gassing people driven into underground refuges.

Location

Each location that was attacked was chosen for strategic purposes. Khan Sheikhoun was a rebel and jihadist stronghold. Khanal-Assal was a highly contested area between government and opposition forces which had been fought over for weeks. Ghouta was within a rebel weapons supply route from Jordan and was a centre of sustained fighting. Halabja, Northern Iraq, harboured groups whom the Iraqis aimed to kill or terrorise—Iranians attempting to occupy the city of Sulaymaniyah, Iranian forces, pro-Iranian Kurds and civilians (BBC News, 25 January 2010).

Perpetrator–Victim Relationship

In the Khan Sheikhoun attack, the direct perpetrators were the forces of President Assad. Intended victims were the 'rebel fighters' and jihadists linked to al-Qaeda who largely controlled the Idib Province (BBC, April 2017).

Regarding Khanal-Assal, both the Syrian government and opposition accused each other of carrying out the attack (BBC News, 19 March 2013a). Victims—men, women, and children—were civilians and government soldiers (Barnard 2013). Because wind carried the gas to a neighbourhood near the proposed attack site, different claims could be made. The attack was perpetrated either by the opposition to deliberately kill government forces or by government forces unintentionally killing their own. A Free Syrian Army spokesperson claimed that the government attacked its own people to smear the opposition (TIME 2013).

If Syrian forces were responsible for the chemical attack on Eastern Ghouta, the target would be the Syrian opposition controlling the area. In Halabja, Northern Iraq, Iraqi forces attacked the city killing Kurds, and members of the Iran armed forces.

As might be expected in warfare, the perpetrators and victims are generally groups of people whose loyalties are opposed to each other. Also, perpetrators may be defined ethnically (as with the Kurds) and considered a threat to the regime. In the confusion of warfare, the victims are not always the ones targeted.

Conclusion

Situational Crime Prevention

Warfare by its nature scuppers or limits attempts at prevention. Specific attacks having taken place have by definition largely evaded prevention. However, we can see in them opportunities for mitigation that have been taken or missed.

Control tools/weapons through international agreements and inspections may be constrained in a civil war. Territorial boundaries are porous, various factions may have secret access to chemical weapons, and an accurate picture is evasive. However, even where whole state entities are in conflict, control of chemical weapons can be difficult. *Target hardening* can include using protective items and related survival training where time and resources permit. It is characteristic of war that weapons are not controllable by the opposition or by would-be peacemakers and that targets, especially civilians, are difficult to 'harden'. Chemical weapons are especially difficult for civilians to protect themselves against. Poison can inflict short- and long-term damage and works silently creating anxiety and fear among military personnel and civilians.

Surveillance evidence can include witness reports and camera recordings. Autopsy evidence and environmental samples of poisons offer supporting evidence. With more formal surveillance, investigational remit disputes between governments and inspectors can delay access to sites. If evidence of chemical weapons use is found, different sides can form different interpretations. Where those responsible are eventually punished, this is expected to deter others by demonstrating an increased risk.

Where there are planned bombing raids on known areas, it may be possible to *conceal targets* where intelligence is available. Even then, the chance outcome of some chemical attacks can annul preventive measures. Targeted people may think that they are concealed underground but may still be vulnerable.

Within a war zone, *avoiding disputes* can involve providing safe zones, or separate areas for opposing factions. To *reduce emotional arousal* implies softening war rhetoric. International pressure can de-escalate the conflict and neutral countries can provide a forum for combatants to seek a peaceful resolution. This is hindered where factions differ about who is responsible for an attack.

In wartime, *setting rules* suggests citing internationally agreed codes of conduct and providing evidence that they were broken, so challenging perpetrators' excuses. Sometimes 'rules' delineating crimes against humanity eventually lead to perpetrators being held accountable.

Means, Motive, Opportunity, Location, and Perpetrator–Victim Relationship

The *means* of killing in chemical warfare—chemical agents—attracts abhorrence reflected in specific conventions and related inspection regimes. This may relate to the power of chemical weapons to inspire terror. Such poisons can cause lingering death affecting the morale of surviving troops and terrifying civilians. Some hard-to-detect colourless and odourless poisonous agents make precautions especially difficult to implement.

The *motives* in warfare for using chemical weapons are to defeat or weaken opposing forces, and to demoralise troops and civilians. The motives are in fact like those relating to other weapons in warfare. *Opportunity* to use chemical weapons includes minimising the risk by initiating an early-morning or night-time raid. Using rockets to deliver chemical agents reduces the risk to the perpetrators compared with deploying piloted aircraft. Chemical agents can be sprayed to cover a wide area. Pre-bombardment can drive people underground before using heavier-than-air poison gas. *Locations* are attacked for strategic purposes as an enemy stronghold, a highly contested area, or an enemy weapons supply route.

In wartime, participants are enemies fighting over territory, or seeking revenge for previous attack on their own forces, or carrying out some form of 'ethnic cleansing' (usually related to territory). Victims can be men, women, and children, civilians, or military personnel. Accusations may be made that one side is killing its own forces to smear the opposition and set up revenge attacks. *Perpetrators and victims* of conflict are generally groups with opposing loyalties or who are defined ethnically and considered a threat to the regime.

Suggested Activities

Consult the Congressional Research Service website (www.crs.gov) and read the report on chemical weapons (Shea 2013).

List the weapons described according to their likely effectiveness in warfare and military conflict from the more to the least 'effective'. Qualify your judgement as necessary according to the conditions in which the chemical agent is deployed.

Key Texts

Bunker, R. J. (2019) *Contemporary Chemical Weapon Use in Syria and Iraq by the Assad Regime and the Islamic State* Carlisle Barrack, PA, Strategic Studies Institute and the United States Army War College Press (February 2019) https://ssi.armywarcollege.edu/pubs/display.cfm?pubID=1400 see the site's PDF download.
This monograph outlines chemical weapons capabilities and the contemporary use of chemical weapons in Syria and Iraq. It suggests considerations for the US army when a land force operates in a contaminated area, or confronts opponents having chemical weapons.
Bentley, M. (2016) *Syria and the Chemical Weapons Taboo: Exploiting the Forbidden* (New Approaches to Conflict Analysis) Manchester, UK, Manchester University Press.
This book, informed by conflict analysis, suggests that seeing chemical weapons as 'taboo' can have unintended negative consequences.

References

Barnard, A. (2013, March 19). Syria and Activists Trade Charges on Chemical Weapons. *New York Times*. www.nytimes.com/2013/03/20/world/middleeast/syria-developments.html?pagewanted=all.

BBC News. (2010, January 25). "Chemical Ali' Executed in Iraq After Halabja ruling' BBC.

BBC News. (2013a, March 19). Syrians Trade Khan al-Hassal Chemical Weapons Claims. https://www.bbc.co.uk/news/world-middle-east-21841217.

BBC News. (2013b, August 27). Syria Crisis: Russia and China Step Up Warning Over Strike. https://www.bbc.co.uk/news/world-us-canada-23845800.

BBC News. (2017, April 26). Syria Chemical Attack – What We Know. www.bbc.co.uk/news/world-middle-east-39500947.

BBC On This Day. (1988, March 16). 1988 thousands die in Halabja gas attack' BBC.

Blomfield, A. (2010, January 25). Chemical Ali Executed in Iraq. *The Telegraph*. https://www.telegraph.co.uk/news/worldnews/middleeast/iraq/7072687/Chemical-Ali-executed-in-Iraq.html.

Cambridge University Press. (2019). https://dictionary.cambridge.org/dictionary/english/warfare.

Chairman of the Joint Intelligence Committee, Joint Intelligence Organisation. (2013, August 29). *Syria: Reported Chemical Weapons Use – Letter form the Chairman of the Joint Intelligence Committee* London, Cabinet Office. www.gov.uk/government/publications/syria-reported-chemical-weapons-use-joint-intelligence-committee-letter; https://assets.publishing.service.gov.uk/government/uploads/system/uploads/attachment_data/file/235094/Jp_115_JD_PM_Syria_Reported_Chemical_Weapon_Use_with_annex.pdf.

de Bretton-Gordon, H. (2016, March 16). Remembering Halabja Chemical Attack. *Al Jazeera*. https://www.aljazeera.com/indepth/opinion/2016/03/remembering-halabja-chemical-attack-160316061221074.html.

Del Boca, A. (1969). *The Ethiopian War, 1935–1941* (Trans. from the Italian by P. D. Cummins). Chicago, IL: University of Chicago Press.

Dickinson, E. (2013, September 9). Arab League Says Assad Crossed 'Global Red Line' with Chemical Attack. *The National*. https://web.archive.org/web/20130920012715/http://www.thenational.ae/news/world/middle-east/arab-league-says-assad-crossed-global-red-line-with-chemical-attack.

Dupuy, R. E., & Dupuy, T. N. (2007 [1991]). *The Collins Encyclopaedia of Military History from 3500 B.C. to the Present* BCA/Harper Collins.

Edmonds, J. E. (1993 [1932]). *Military Operations France and Belgium, 1916* (History of the Great War Based on Official Documents by Direction of the Historical Section of the Committee of Imperial Defence) London: Macmillan.

Ellison, D. H. (2007). *Handbook of Chemical and Biological Warfare Agents* (2nd ed.). Boca Raton, FL: CRC Press.

Grip, L., & Hart, H. (2009, October). The Use of Chemical Weapons in the 1935–36 Italo-Ethiopian War. *SIPRI Arms Control and Non-proliferation*

Programme. Stockholm, Stockholm International Peace Research Institute. https://www.sipri.org/sites/default/files/Italo-Ethiopian-war.pdf.

Heller, C. E. (1984, September). *Chemical Warfare in World War I: The American Experience, 1917–1918* US Army Command and General Staff College.

Hiltermann, J. R. (2007). *A Poisonous Affair: America, Iraq, and the Gassing of Halabja*. New York: Cambridge University Press.

Hubbard, B., Mazzetti, M., & Landler, M. (2013, August 26). Blasts in the Night, a Smell, and a Flood of Syrian Victims. *The New York Times*.

Human Rights Watch. (2013, September 10). Attacks on Ghouta – Analysis of Alleged Use of Chemical Weapons in Syria. https://www.hrw.org/report/2013/09/10/attacks-ghouta/analysis-alleged-use-of-chemical-weapons-syria#.

League of Nations, Letter. (1936). Letter 13 April 1936, from the Ethiopian Representative to the Secretary-General, 13 April 1936, *League of Nations Official Journal* Annex 1592, April 1936, pp. 479–80.

National Evaluation. (2017, April). Chemical Attack on 4 April 2017 Khan Sheikhoun – Clandestine Syrian Chemical Weapons Programme. https://www.diplomatie.gouv.fr/IMG/pdf/170425_-_evaluation_nationale_-_anglais_-_final_cle0dbf47-1.pdf.

Notman, N. (2014, June 9). Explosive End for Japan's Second World War Chemical Weapons. Chemistry World (The Royal Society of Chemistry). https://www.chemistryworld.com/news/explosive-end-for-japans-second-world-war-chemical-weapons/7449.article.

Office of the Press Secretary, The White House. (2013, August 30). *Government Assessment of the Syrian Governments Use of Chemical Weapons on August 21, 2013*. https://obamawhitehouse.archives.gov/the-press-office/2013/08/30/government-assessment-syrian-government-s-use-chemical-weapons-august-21.

Organisation for the Prohibition of Chemical Weapons. (2006). *Remembering All Victims of Chemical Warfare* (See www.opcw.org/ and search 'Remembering All Victims of Chemical Warfare' 29 April 2006).

Reuters. (2013, July 9). Russia: Syria Rebels Likely Behind Aleppo Chemical Attack. Reuters.

Rosenfeld, E. (2017, April 6). Trump Launches Attack on Syria with 59 Tomahawk Missiles. CNCC. www.cnbc.com/2017/04/06/us-military-has-launched-more-50-than-missiles-aimed-at-syria-nbc-news.html.

Schneditz, M. (2008). Chemische Kampfstoffe: Geschichte, Entwicklung und Einsatz GRIN Verlag Auflage.

Sellstom, A., Cairns, S., & Barbeschi, M. (2013). *Report of the United Nations Mission to Investigate Allegations of the Use of Chemical Weapons in the Syrian Arab Republic on the Alleged Use of Weapons in the Ghouta Area of Damascus on 21 August 2013* United Nations 16 September 2013.

Shea, D. A. (2013, September 13). *Chemical Weapons: A Summary Report of Characteristics and Effects* Washington, DC, Congressional Research Service 7-5700. www.crs.gov RS42862 and https://fas.org/sgp/crs/nuke/R42862.pdf.

Stepanov, A. A., & Popov, J. N. (1962). Khimicheskoe Oruzhiye i Osnovy Protivokhimicheskoi Zashchity (Chemical weapons and principles of anti-chemical defence) Moscow.

Thomas, F. (2014). *Behind the Gasmask: The US Chemical Warfare Service in War and Peace*. Champaign, IL: University of Illinois Press.

TIME. (2013, April 1). The Mystery Behind a Deadly Chemical Attack. *TIME*.

United Nations. (2013, December 12). *United Nations Mission to Investigate Allegations of the Use of Chemical Weapons in the Syrian Arab Republic – Final Report* United Nations.

United Nations General Assembly Human Rights Council. (2014, February 12). Report of the Independent International Commission of Inquiry on the Syrian Arab Republic. https://www.refworld.org/docid/53182eed4.html.

7

Mass Suicide Using Poison

Introduction

After looking at definitions of mass suicide including by poison, I consider historical instances. Next, two examples of mass suicide by poisoning are described and each analysed in relation to Situational Crime Prevention (SCP). Firstly, I discuss the Heaven's Gate cult in which in 1997, in California, 39 members killed themselves. They took poison and expedited their deaths through suffocation by covering their heads with plastic bags. Secondly, I look at the 1978 mass suicide of over 900 people in Jonestown, Guyana when Rev Jim Jones instructed his followers to poison themselves and their children as an act of supposed revolutionary suicide. I give an overview of the two events through the lens of SCP and consider means, motive, opportunity, location, and perpetrator-victim relationships.

© The Author(s) 2020   **147**
M. Farrell, *Criminology of Poisoning Contexts*,
https://doi.org/10.1007/978-3-030-40830-5_7

Defining Mass Suicide

Etymologically, 'suicide' derives from the Latin 'sui', meaning 'of oneself' and 'cidium' referring to 'killing' as encapsulated in the briefest definitions such as 'the taking of one's own life' (Anderson 2007, p. 1822). More precisely, suicide implies taking one's own life intentionally and voluntarily. This reflects the understanding when in some countries suicide was a crime, but the individual was not criminally culpable if they were unable to act rationally, that is, with intent, for example because of mental disorder. Specifying that suicide is a voluntary act keeps out of the definition instances where someone might be forced to take their own life by another threatening them. Medically, suicide is distinguished from deliberate self-harm (attempted suicide). However, the two are linked in that attempts are one of the indicators of a higher risk of actual suicide (Kumar and Clark 2005, p. 1296).

In mass suicide, there may be debate about the numbers that are involved with some commentators arguing that it needs to be a large group. At a minimum in mass suicide, two or more people kill themselves simultaneously or in close succession. Desperation may be a cause. Thwarted lovers may make a pact to die together. A whole family may commit suicide together under extreme duress. In conflicts, a defeated or near-defeated group may die by their own hands rather than be captured. Mass suicide numbers can be large where religious and quasi-religious groups are involved. Poisoning is sometimes used because individuals may see it as a less-painful way to die than some alternatives.

Mass suicide can involve individuals and groups arranging that others do the killing as part of a pact before ending their own lives as reported at Masada, Israel (Stiebel 2007). Sometimes, in fighting an opponent, a few individuals bring about the deaths of followers with their compliance, as with those resisting French re-enslavement in Guadeloupe (Moitt 1996).

Mass Suicides in History

Historically, mass suicides have involved different means including the sword, burning, explosion, and people casting themselves down from a great height, as well as poisoning.

It is said that in 73 AD over 900 members of Jewish Zealots of the Sicarii community were defending the high refuge of Masada. They took their lives (as a community not individually) rather than surrender to encroaching Roman forces. Each man killed members of his family then men drew lots to kill one another until the last one took his own life (Stiebel 2007). A version of events by Josephus in *The Wars of the Jews* indicates death by the sword, referring to individuals 'offering their necks to the stroke'. Some researchers question accounts of the event.

In 1337, the castle of Pilénai in Lithuania was attacked by Teutonic Knights. Duke Margiris and his followers, recognising defeat, committed suicide and burned the castle to destroy anything of possible value to the enemy (Baronas 2010).

Napoleon, in 1802, reinstated slavery (abolished ten years earlier) in France's Caribbean colonies. Former slaves in Guadeloupe rebelled rather than be re-enslaved. Led by Louis Delgrès, they fought the French army sent to enforce the policy. Looking defeat in the face, in May 1802, at the battle of Matouba, Delgrès and 400 followers ignited their stores of gunpower committing suicide and attempting to simultaneously kill some French troops (Moitt 1996).

In the area of Souli, Greece, in 1803 during the Turkish rule of the country, Ottoman forces held power. Pursued by their enemy, the inhabitants of the district fled to mount Zalongo. To avoid capture, the women threw their children from the summit and then jumped themselves (Sakellariou 1997).

Towards the end of the Warsaw Ghetto uprising, in 1943, many fighters of the ZOB (the Jewish Fighting Organisation) were confined to a hidden shelter beneath a house on Mila 18. Many ingested poison to avoid being captured by the Nazis. Some of the resistance fighters managed to escape the ghetto and join with partisan groups in the forests around the city (the United States Holocaust Memorial Museum, accessed December 2019).

Cults

'Cult' derives from the Latin 'cultus', which has various meanings including 'education' and 'worship' and can be defined in positive and negative terms. It refers to devotion to an intellectual or artistic interest such as a book or a movie as when it is said that a certain new novel has attracted a 'cult following'. More negatively, 'cult' can refer to 'a religion regarded as unorthodox or spurious' (*Merriam-Webster*, accessed December 2019). As well as a religion, the term can refer to belief systems including pagan ones as with the 'cult of Apollo'. 'Cult' also designates the people involved. Those who form part of a cult may be known as 'members', 'adherents', 'disciples', or 'followers'. A cult may have a leader who is seen as charismatic.

At its potentially most sinister, a cult may demand strict adherence to rules and behaviour that erode members' critical thinking and awareness, require members to live in isolation from the rest of society, and insist on obedience to the cult leader.

Situational Crime Prevention

Situational Crime Prevention (SCP) is fully described in the chapter 'Theory and Poison Contexts'. Briefly, five general strategies are each associated with five opportunity-reducing techniques. Regarding the strategy **increase the effort** of perpetrators are the strategies 'target harden', 'control access to facilities', 'screen exits', 'deflect offenders', and 'control tools/weapons'. **Increase the risks** concerns 'extend guardianship', 'assist natural surveillance', 'reduce anonymity', 'utilise place managers', and 'strengthen formal surveillance'. For **reduce rewards** to the perpetrator the techniques are 'conceal targets', 'remove targets', 'identify property', 'disrupt markets', and 'deny benefits'. Techniques to **reduce provocation** comprise 'reduce frustrations and stress', 'avoid disputes', 'reduce emotional arousal', 'neutralise peer pressure', and 'discourage imitation'. **Remove excuses** concerns 'set rules', 'post instructions', 'alert conscience', 'assist compliance', and 'control drugs and alcohol'.

Heaven's Gate

Applewhite Meets Nettles

Son of a Texan Presbyterian minister, Marshall Applewhite began ministry training but switched to music. Unable to make it performing, Applewhite settled for teaching. In 1968, after 16 years of marriage, and two children, he divorced. By 1972, Applewhite had psychological problems, and his university career was precarious. Then he received a life-transforming message from 'the Lord' that entities previously considered angels were UFOs.

Born in 1927, Bonnie Nettles was raised a Baptist in Houston and qualified as a registered nurse. Aged 22, she married and subsequently had three children. Her marriage was dissolved in 1972. Developing occult beliefs, she conducted home seances, and consulted fortune tellers prophesying she would meet a mysterious man.

The pair met in March 1972. Nettles did astrological readings finding alignment between Applewhite's stars and her own. Applewhite recognised her ability to understand his divinations. They took to the road on New Year's Day 1973, Nettles's leaving her three young children with their father (Bearak 1997).

Their Mission

After months travelling in 1973, the two shared a platonic bond and a desire to escape life 'alive'. Beside the Rogue River, Oregon, they became convinced that God had given them a mission. They continued travelling North America, camping, taking menial jobs, and sharing their message at churches or religious bookstores. But finding people uninspired, they reworked their beliefs. God required unconditional love of Him alone implying renunciation of wealth, family, and sensual desires. They must lead others to a higher level. Both would soon be killed by the unfaithful but, regaining life days later, would ascend in a cloud. The Lord would then destroy the world.

In May 1974, in Houston, Applewhite and Nettles (later known among other titles as 'The Two') recruited their first disciple, realtor Sharon Morgan, caught in an unhappy marriage. Six days later, she left her husband and two young daughters. On the road, Sharon visited occult bookstores and metaphysical centers, meeting people, and asking some if they would like to hear The Two's message. After only a month, guilt ridden about leaving her children, Sharon looked forward to stopping in Dallas, to visit an old companion. In fact, the friend had alerted Sharon's husband, who seized Sharon and brought her home.

Soon after, a routine police check showed Applewhite had stolen a vehicle during travels across America. Jailed for six months, Applewhite wrote a creed shared with Nettles. People must experience a chrysalis stage prior to life in the Next Level. Applewhite and Nettles would teach their doctrine. A validation would soon come, when The Two would be killed, then resurrected in a cloud of light (Bearak 1997).

Followers Are Recruited

After Applewhite had served his jail term, The Two went to California, where they contacted churches and spiritual centres. One meeting in May 1975 at the Los Angeles home of a psychic recruited two dozen people, keen on taking a spaceship to heaven. The Two took their followers to their Rogue River revelation spot, announcing that the arrival of the prophesied spaceship was imminent. Days later, the flock was sent out in pairs as missionaries across America, penniless but allowed to ask for charity. They reconvened two months later in a Wyoming campground.

The leaders arranged meetings in school auditoria. Although The Two avoided talking about spaceships now, their followers did not. A meeting in September 1975, in Waldport, Oregon recruited 20 new disciples to the 'UFO cult'. Stories of 'disappearing' followers made national news, driving Applewhite and Nettles into hiding.

The Two sent their followers on more road trips, secretly communicating via post office boxes and relayed phone messages. Members reunited in June 1976, in a National Forest in Wyoming. The Two now weaned out members smoking marijuana or having sex, which were forbidden, and announced that the 'demonstration' of their death and resurrection was postponed. With now around 70 disciples, they started a special class. The Two had no individual memories of their lives on the Next Level, as knowledge reached them via psychic communication from 'the fathers'. Everyone had one older member as a guide. Nettles was Applewhite's 'father' in a series of links leading to a chief of chiefs.

Between 1976 and 1979, the group moved seasonally between camping in the Rockies and Texas, living off a few members' personal wealth. They aimed to constrain a sense of self by distrusting one's judgement, limiting curiosity, and eschewing attention. Partners were assigned, each watching the other's obedience to a strict regimen, although there were also leisure activities. At night, teams sought signs of their spaceship (Bearak 1997).

Temptations

In 1979, the group moved into several houses, in Denver and the Southwest. Worried about being tracked down by authorities or broken families, The Two kept the group moving.

By 1981, some members took menial jobs to help finances. They put in fictionalised applications and drove without licenses. Later, using their real names they took better jobs suiting their skills, but still offered false documents. Members left for work with pocket money which all had to be accounted for. Those without jobs worked in the houses, each day following precisely scheduled procedures. Seats were assigned for class sessions, even for watching television. Sex being forbidden, heterosexuals slept with the same sex, homosexuals with the opposite sex. Violators had to announce their lapses publicly. The most sex-beset individuals pressed Applewhite (unsuccessfully) to allow them to be castrated.

Nettles developed cancer and, in the summer of 1985, under an alias, died in Parkland Hospital, Dallas. Applewhite explained her 'leftover body' by a notion of a parallel body with a different molecular structure. This grew as one mastered knowledge of the Next Level in preparation for heaven (Bearak 1997).

A New Start

In 1988, Applewhite felt that his Next Level fathers wanted the prophe-cies spread. The group mailed New Age centres. Applewhite again spoke of the move to the Next Level growing near. This age was ending, Lucifer controlled the earth, and humans must perish. Four years later, the group, then living in Laguna Hills, California, broadcast homemade videotapes. Later, in newspapers worldwide the group promised to respond to anyone interested in the 'final offer'. The class was now about 25. Applewhite finally reconsidered earlier requests and he and seven others were castrated.

In 1994, the group sold most of its possessions except transportation and computers and split into four evangelical teams, travelling in a 'last chance' cross-country proselytising effort. After nine months of travel-ling, group membership reached 45. Lacking the 'demonstration' of his murder and ascent, Applewhite considered death requiring no outsiders. In September 1994, near San Clemente, California, he called a meeting to discuss suicide and potions to make it painless.

The following year, astronomers sighted the Comet Hale-Bopp. Someone had photographed a spot of light rumoured to be a spaceship in tow. By fall 1996, the group was running a computer-consulting business and living in a gated estate in Rancho Santa Fe, California. Mass suicide now offered members hope. Applewhite was 65 and might leave them, but through suicide they could evade mortality by being transported to the spaceship. They prepared farewell videos (Bearak 1997).

On 26 March 1997, the bodies of 39 members were found. They had killed themselves in three waves from 24th through 26th March. Survivors arranged their dead comrades' bodies before killing themselves. Each wore sports clothing and Heaven's Gate armbands. Most lay on their beds draped in a purple cloth. Each had pocket money, and beside them packed luggage. They had consumed poisonous levels of phenobarbital and drunk vodka. A few had tied plastic bags on their heads to asphyxiate themselves (Zennie 2012).

Heaven's Gate and SCP

In the Heaven's Gate cult, the lead perpetrators were Marshall Applewhite and (before her death) Bonnie Nettles. Given their suicides, cult members were in a sense both perpetrators and victims. They took their lives apparently voluntarily and intentionally. However, the extent to which by the time of their deaths they were indoctrinated or responsible for their actions is open to question. In considering techniques concerning perpetrators, we therefore look at both leader and followers.

Regarding **increasing the effort** of perpetrators, *hardening targets* concerns intervening at some point during the events leading to the suicides. If members are targets for recruitment to a group in whose membership they die, what preventive actions are possible? Educational bodies and others can make potential converts aware of ways that cults can undermine their critical scrutiny. Such attempts may be weakened where people are willing to be convinced and are vulnerable. *Controlling tools/ weapons* involves authorities restricting access to poisons generally (including ones that might be used for suicide). However, once an individual or a group decide that they will take their own lives, even where many poisons are legally restricted, prevention is difficult. Other more accessible poisons can be found, or other non-poison methods of suicide may be used.

Turning to **increasing the risks** for perpetrators, *reducing the anonymity* of cult leaders and their practices can make them less convincing. Hence the evasiveness and reticence of leaders (and some followers) to face public scrutiny. In the autumn of 1975, when The Two took their message to Chicago, the story became national news. Some followers welcomed publicity thinking that as prophesied The Two would be killed and ascend to heaven, but in contrast the Two went into hiding. *Assisting natural surveillance* suggests supporting any group member who has second thoughts and wants to leave, and perhaps wishes to report unlawful or suspect activities. Relatedly, *strengthening formal surveillance* applies to authorities getting inside information on the group's activities so that they can step in where a law is broken. A meeting in September 1975, at a motel in Oregon, recruited 20 new disciples. Worried relatives and friends called police and hired detectives, and journalists began to investigate but seemingly with little effect.

Reducing rewards for perpetrators by *removing targets* can involve authorities taking an individual away from a cult perhaps to a refuge. This might especially apply with those who are vulnerable and otherwise unprotected, like minors or abused individuals. Given that disciple Sharon Morgan was recovered by her husband, clearly one way of removing targets is through relatives and friends intervening. This may have been viable even for the 1996 suicides in California. However, by that time (and before) The Two evaded possible attempts to remove followers by being secretive and highly security conscious. When they sent their members on road trips, The Two communicated with them secretly. The group kept moving to avoid scrutiny from concerned families or the authorities or lived in houses in various locations. When taking work outside the group, members faked documentation. *Disrupting markets* can refer to pressure groups monitoring websites or advertisements which recruit cult group members and requesting authorities to intervene where there are concerns. To avoid this, The Two had their own sources of recruitment. Heaven's Gate contacted existing groups interested in esoteric beliefs, mailed fliers to churches and spiritual centres, and held a recruitment meeting at the Los Angeles home of a psychic.

Turning to **reduce provocation**, *neutralising peer pressure* can involve raising awareness of the potential harm of cult membership. It includes being alert to injunctions discouraging critical or independent thinking. In Heaven's Gate, rules were devised such as at the camp training encouraging members to distrust their own judgement, avoid inappropriate curiosity, and shun attention seeking. A strict regimen, detailed scheduling and procedures, and public and private confession were enforced.

Concerning **removing excuses**, none of the techniques seem to apply to Heaven's Gate.

The Jonestown Massacre

Events surrounding the Jonestown massacre took place at a time in America when cults, off-beat churches, communes, and other social experiments were popular. Some were a positive force or at least harmless, while others had sinister undercurrents. The People's Temple Agricultural Project or 'Jonestown' in the jungle of North Western Guyana, South America was named after Reverend Jim Jones. He was a charismatic but paranoid cult leader who persuaded his followers to commit mass suicide by poisoning. Over 900 people died on 18 November 1978, including 300 who were 17 years old or younger. They were followers of the People's Temple of the Disciples of Christ.

Jones's Early Life and the Development of the People's Temple

Jones grew up in poverty in Indiana during the Great Depression. He was described as an 'intelligent and strange' child (Conroy 2018). In adulthood, Jones developed an interest in communism, anti-racism, and reducing poverty. He was also drawn to charismatic movements in Christianity.

Jones formed the group that was to become known as the People's Temple in 1956 in Indianapolis. Its stance against racism initially drew in many African Americans. In 1960, the congregation affiliated with another group, the Disciples of Christ. Four years later, Jones was ordained into that church. In the mid-1960s, the group moved to Redwood Valley California. Jones developed good relationships with sections of the press and some local politicians. By 1971 when the church had transferred to San Francisco, members were expected to hand over their personal wealth and work long hours unpaid. They sometimes broke contact with their families and were expected to bring up their children in the commune. There were reports that, to demonstrate their commitment, they were asked to sign testimonials that they had molested their children and that the church retained these documents for potential future blackmail (Conroy 2018).

Jones developed an increasingly overblown perception of his importance suggesting sometimes that if followers wanted to see him as a god,
then he would comply. He had an ambition, spurred on by growing distrust of US authorities of establishing a church outside of the United
States and beyond its interfering jurisdiction. Believing that the United
States was in danger of nuclear holocaust, he searched for somewhere
where his church would be sheltered. He chose Guyana with its sympa-
thetic socialist regime.

Founding Jonestown

In 1973, Jones leased land from the Guyanese government to convert
into an agricultural settlement. Development was slow so that by 1977
there were still only about 50 people living there. They moved to the
jungle site seeking to form a utopia in which individuals of all races and
ages lived together as a family with common ownership of goods and in
total equality. Jones remained resident in the United States.

Jones Moves to the Guyana Settlement

As a printed exposé of some of the problems with the People's Temple was
about to be published, Jones and several hundred followers left the United
States for Guyana and the Jonestown compound.

The influx created problems. The place was overcrowded. Members
were segregated by gender so married couples had to live apart. People
were expected to work long hours and some became sick in the heat and
humidity. While many liked the settlement, some wanted to leave.
However, the compound was very isolated in the middle of jungle and
circled by armed guards. Members also needed Jones's permission to
leave the site.

Visit from Congressman Ryan

Some former members and the relatives of current members were uneasy about this move into isolation. They pressed for investigation, and this led on 17 November 1978 to Democratic Congressmen Leo Ryan of San Mateo, California, visiting the site. With him were an adviser, a television crew, and worried relatives of cult members.

The following day, as Ryan's party were leaving, several of the residents requested to go with them. Jones became agitated at these requests and one of his followers attacked Ryan with a knife. Unharmed, the congressman left the compound.

However, Jones then instructed some of his followers to ambush and kill Ryan at the airstrip from which he and his party were planning to depart. Ryan and four others were duly murdered as they tried to board their aircraft.

The Mass Suicide

Meanwhile, in the compound, Jones ordered everyone to gather in the pavilion. Informing members of the impending plan to kill Ryan and his group, he explained that once this was done, the community would no longer be safe. In retribution, US forces would soon attack them. The only escape was to commit an act of 'revolutionary suicide'. When news came that Ryan was indeed dead, Jones became more urgent. Poison had been prepared comprising cyanide, sedatives, and fruit juices. Followers were told to kill their children first, using syringes as necessary to deposit poison into the mouths of babies. Members then poisoned themselves. A few escaped into the jungle or hid in corners of the compound. In one bizarre twist, an elderly woman appears to have slept through the whole incident and woke to find everyone dead.

When news of the events began to leak out, the military entered Jonestown to find numerous corpses lying on the ground beginning to decompose in the jungle heat. The US Army reported that 909 bodies were recovered from Jonestown, excluding people killed at the airstrip (Moore 2019). The vast majority had seemingly killed themselves. A few including Jim Jones had bullet wounds. Some were injected with cyanide, although it was unclear whether this had been voluntarily or forcibly administered. Some had taken cyanide orally and had also had injections suggesting that this might have been to speed up the deaths (Luther 2018; Conroy 2018).

Fondakowski (2013) brings together accounts of those who were involved with Jonestown.

Among filmed reports and documentaries about the People's Temple is *Jonestown: The Life and death of People's Temple* (https://www.youtube.com/watch?v=sOqszjh_9es).

Jonestown and SCP

In the Jonestown suicides, viewed as a criminal activity, Jones and his closest followers effectively perpetrated the killings (Reiterman and Jacobs 2008 e.g. pxi). Firstly, the deaths would likely not have taken place had not Jones ordered them. Secondly, with babies and very young children who constituted a sizable minority of the deaths, parents carried out the killing under the direction of Jim Jones. Thirdly, it is reported that armed guards surrounding the commune acted as agents of coercion when members killed themselves.

Increasing the effort of perpetrators by *hardening targets* implies making it more difficult for perpetrators to influence and isolate potential followers. In retrospect, the best opportunity for authorities to act to harden targets may have been before the plans to develop a site in Guyana. This was the time that Jones was planning and carrying out his project to establish a compound outside the United States beyond US government influence. He leased the land in Guyana in 1973, and even by 1975 only about 50 members were involved in preparing it for occupation. During this period, and certainly when Jones precipitately moved to the remote site with many more followers, it would have been opportune to discourage or prevent followers travelling there. Indeed, some relatives pressed to have the commune investigated leading to Ryan's visit. *Controlling tools/ weapons* by preventing access to poisons involved in the suicides was avoided because the settlement was isolated, inaccessible, and outside direct US legal jurisdiction.

Concerning **increasing the risks** to perpetrators, *reducing anonymity* applies to exposing a cult and its leaders where there are concerns, for example by releasing negative publicity. In Jonestown, the threat of such exposure precipitated the move to Guyana to escape accountability. It led to congressional interest but inadvertently moved cult members towards further danger. *Assisting natural surveillance* suggests supporting cult members wanting to get out. Ryan finding that some group members indeed wished to leave attempted to facilitate this. His visit also represented *strengthening formal surveillance* but in the event was ineffective.

Reducing rewards to the perpetrator by *removing targets* can apply to authorities taking an individual from the cult group. Ryan's attempt to take away members on visiting Jonestown failed because of its isolation and Jones's determination to resist. *Disrupting markets* can involve pressure groups monitoring media advertisements which recruit cult members and requesting authorities to intervene. Because the People's Temple had once been a respected organisation supported by local politicians and the wider community, there seemed at first no need to disrupt recruitment of members. Yet over time, Jones's behaviour including his self-aggrandisement and paranoia alerted authorities. Also, in retrospect, reports of members being abused might have been acted upon earlier or more vigorously. Such intervention was inhibited by the initial respectability of the group and the enforcement of members' loyalty.

Turning to **reducing provocations**, 'neutralising peer pressure' applies to raising awareness of the possible harm of cult membership among recruits or existing members who might be drawn into criminal or foolhardy acts. It can include alerting individuals to cult rules, discouraging critical or independent thinking or helping members recognise that they are effectively being held against their will. When Jones finally ordered members to commit suicide, there was a vain attempt to resist from at least one woman, but it was too late.

Concerning **remove excuses** none of the techniques seem to apply.

Overview of SCP and Mass Suicide Cults

Techniques to Increase the Effort of Perpetrators

Target hardening of cult members can involve relatives and friends intervening and sometimes forcibly removing them. Heaven's gate disciple Sharon Morgan was recovered by her husband. Similar interventions prior to the 1996 suicides were rendered less likely by the group's heightened security. With Jonestown, opportunities for intervention by relatives and authorities arose when Jones started to lease land in Guyana and when he precipitately moved to the remote site with many more followers. Some relatives pressed for Ryan to investigate the commune, but it proved too late. Targets are also hardened where cult ideas are publicised and scrutinised, making potential converts aware of strategies undermining their critical scrutiny. Such preventive strategies are weakened where people are gullible or vulnerable.

Controlling tools/weapons applies to limiting access to poisons that may be used for suicide (or homicide). Heaven's Gate sidestepped this because members seemingly agreed the suicides, and voluntarily acquired and used poison. Jonestown evaded this preventive measure through its isolation and inaccessibility.

Techniques to Increase the Risks to Perpetrators

To *reduce anonymity* of cult leaders and their practices, opponents can encourage public scrutiny, air negative publicity, and challenge the cult's message. Leaders can dodge this by going into hiding, or it can even be counterproductive. When Heaven's Gate attracted national news interest., the principals went underground. With Jonestown, the threat of exposure precipitated the full-scale move to Guyana, inadvertently further endangering cult members.

Assisting natural surveillance suggests supporting a group member wanting to leave or reporting inappropriate activities. With Heaven's Gate, this occurred occasionally. In Jonestown, Ryan recognised that some group members were being held forcibly and attempted to free them.

Relatedly *strengthening formal surveillance* applies to investigation or undercover work enabling authorities to intervene if necessary. Following a Heaven's Gate recruitment meeting in Oregon, relatives and friends alerted police, private detectives, and journalists but with limited effect. In Jonestown, Ryan's visit attempting to support whistle-blowers also represented *strengthening formal surveillance*.

Techniques That Reduce Rewards to the Perpetrator

Removing targets can apply to concerned families or authorities taking an individual from a cult. After Sharon Morgan's removal, Heaven's Gate evaded further attempts by arranging secret communications with members, moving to different locations, and creating fake identities. In Jonestown, Ryan's attempt to remove people failed because of resistance and the settlement's isolation.

Disrupting markets can involve pressure groups monitoring websites or advertisements recruiting cult group members and requesting authorities to intervene. To avoid this, Heaven's Gate recruitment involved directly contacting others interested in esoteric beliefs and arranging meetings in private homes. Jim Jones avoided disruption to his recruitment of followers because of the group's initial respectability and the ever-tighter enforcement of members' loyalty.

Reduce Provocations

Neutralising peer pressure can refer to authorities and relatives ensuring that recruits are aware of the potential harm of membership. In Heaven's Gate, camp training rules aimed to limit members' sense of self aided by detailed daily schedules and procedures, and confessions. Regarding Jonestown, peer pressure and coercion was so high that when Jones ordered the mass suicide, members were unable to resist.

Remove Excuses

Concerning removing excuses, none of the techniques seem to apply to cults and potential doomsday suicide pacts such as Heaven's Gate and Jonestown.

Means, Motive, Opportunity, Location, and Perpetrator–Victim Relationship

Means

As the means of killing, Heaven's Gate members took poisonous amounts of phenobarbital in food and drank vodka, then some tied plastic bags on their heads to asphyxiate themselves and expedite death (Zennie 2012). At Jonestown, almost all members took a mixture of cyanide, sedatives, and fruit juice, killing their children first, then poisoning themselves (Luther 2018; Conroy 2018). In both cults, the choice of poison and other substances was to try to ensure speedy death without excessive suffering. Heaven's Gate members took alcohol and expedited their death by asphyxiation, while Jonestown members took sedatives.

Motive

Two aspects can drive cult suicides. Firstly, there are the motives of the cult leaders encouraging or demanding suicide. Also important are the driving forces of cult members who in different degrees take responsibility for their own deaths and sometimes those of others.

Applewhite was the sole leader of Heaven's Gate when suicide developed as the group's destiny. His motive appears to have been following the cult's mission and the guidance that he believed he was receiving from a higher power. Followers seem to have been influenced to take their own lives by a belief in Applewhite and his revelations. In both cases, the driving force was a strong belief that mass suicide would enable members to escape mortality and be transported to a spaceship as an entry to heaven (Zennie 2012).

Jim Jones seems to have been initially motivated by hopes of social justice but over time changed to be driven by paranoia and a desire to control members. His own suicide seems to have been precipitated by a desire to escape the consequences of his involvement in Ryan's murder. He ordered the mass suicide of members in the apparent belief that once the congressman's killing became known, the US government would have the commune destroyed. Evading this was to him an act of 'revolutionary suicide'. Some members killed their own children before killing themselves, which constitutes murder rather than suicide. But the motive for killing others and themselves seems to have been to escape the prospect of being destroyed by others from the outside. They were faced with this as a fait accompli because of the actions of Jones and a few others in murdering Ryan. Underpinning their compliance was a willingness to believe Jones and to follow what he ordered and perhaps reflecting the groups Christian origins, a belief in an afterlife (Luther 2018; Conroy 2018).

Opportunity

Opportunity for mass suicides in cults is provided by the isolation often associated with them and relates to location which we will discuss next.

Heaven's Gate members were separated in a gated community having previously avoided discovery by their relatives or others by various means. This gave the uninterrupted opportunity for suicide of members over several days. Jonestown members were even more isolated, giving more than enough opportunity for suicide. It allowed Jones to exert pressure on members to comply with his orders for a supposed revolutionary gesture.

Location

Location tends to be a key aspect of the cult suicides. Isolation and separation from contact with others who might subvert the cult message is influential. For Heaven's Gate, their final location was a gated community; for Jonestown, it was a remote jungle commune.

Perpetrator–Victim Relationship

In cult mass suicides, leaders are perpetrators in persuading or indoctrinating members to take their own lives. Cult members themselves are both victims of the warped beliefs of the leaders and perpetrators of their own deaths.

As perpetrator, Applewhite was 65 years old, male, Caucasian, middle class and well educated musically (Bearak 1997). Heaven's Gate members who committed suicide in California ranged in age from 26 to 72 years (Zennie 2012). The group comprised 21 men and 18 women, although, sex being forbidden, no children. Some of the group were homosexual as indicated by sleeping arrangements made earlier in the campsite period. A few had themselves castrated (Bearak 1997). Some members were African American, while others were white Caucasian. Members were typically able to generate incomes with a variety of skills and occupations including in computing. None of these demographic features appear to be decisive in the membership. A common thread of membership, given the way they were recruited was an initial tendency to believe in the esoteric and in some form of possible afterlife.

Jim Jones as perpetrator was white, male, and aged 47 years. His education was such that he was ordained by the Independent Assemblies of God (1956) and by the Disciples of Christ (1964). As the US Army reported, 909 bodies were recovered from Jonestown, excluding people killed at the airstrip (Moore 2019). They were men, women, and children. A third were 17 or under and some were babies and young children (Eldridge n.d.). Nearly three-quarters of residents who died at Jonestown were African American (Moore 2019), seemingly reflecting Jones's early church work which attracted many of this group. Most residents were African American women. The occupations of individuals before they moved to Jonestown indicated that they came from working-class and professional backgrounds. At least 27 who died had worked in the US Civil Service. Twenty-one of the dead were military veterans (Moore 2019).

Conclusion

Situational Crime Prevention

With mass suicides that have evaded prevention, one can retrospectively consider steps that might have been taken. *Target hardening* of cult members can involve relatives and friends removing them or encouraging authorities to investigate, but this is hindered where groups heighten security. Cult ideas can be publicised and scrutinised, and potential recruits made aware of coercive techniques, but this may fail where people are gullible or vulnerable. *Controlling tools/weapons* applies to limiting access to poisons, but members may endorse suicide, and may seemingly voluntarily acquire and use poison, and the cult location may be isolated.

Authorities can *reduce the anonymity* of cult practices by encouraging public scrutiny, airing negative publicity, and challenging the cult's message. In response, cult members may go into hiding. *Assisting natural surveillance* suggests supporting a group member in escaping or whistle-blowing. Relatedly *strengthening formal surveillance* involves investigation or undercover work enabling authorities to intervene if necessary, but is weakened if cult members are committed to remaining.

Removing targets (members) from a cult can be thwarted by heightened security, communicating secretly, using false documentation, and staying in remote locations. *Disrupting markets* can involve opponents monitoring cult recruitment communications and alerting authorities, but can be avoided where the cult meets in private venues, has initial respectability, and enforces members' loyalty.

Neutralising peer pressure can involve opponents alerting recruits to the potential harm of membership, making them aware of cult procedures that erode critical thinking, but is evaded where the cult remotely located and members are indoctrinated.

Means, Motive, Opportunity, Location, and Perpetrator–Victim Relationships

Using poison as the *means* of killing in cults aims to ensure speedy death without excessive suffering, or alarming bloodshed. Additional means may be used to accelerate death or make it less distressing.

Cult leaders may be *motivated* by following guidance supposed to be from a higher power. They may be driven by hopes of social justice gradually corrupted by paranoia and a desire to control. Their suicide may be to escape punishment for crimes. Followers may be motivated to take their own lives by belief in the cult leader and their revelations, or an indoctrinated sense that they must obey the leader's orders. They may think they are resisting to malign authorities. Leaders and followers may believe that mass suicide offers entry to a heavenly afterlife.

Opportunity for mass suicides in cults can be provided by the isolation of the members from the rest of society, which also contributes to the capacity of leaders to exert control.

The *location* of cult suicides tends to be isolated so that there is little or no contact with others who might subvert the cult message.

Cult leaders are *perpetrators* in leading members to suicide. Disciples can be both *victims* of the beliefs of leaders and *perpetrators* of their own deaths. Demographic details of leaders—age, sex, ethnicity, social, and educational background—may be less influential than other factors. Key features are mental disorder and firm conviction leading ultimately to corruption of rational thinking and power seeking. Other aspects are the convincing exposition of beliefs. Demographics of followers may reflect the group's aims and values. A cult forbidding sex is unlikely to have child members. One espousing racial equality may well have increased numbers from minority ethnic groups. Where a group lives together, sustaining itself for long periods, members will likely have a variety of skills and occupations. A common thread of membership, given how members are recruited, is an initial interest in the spiritual or esoteric and belief in a possible afterlife.

Suggested Activities

Identify similarities and differences between the Heaven's Gate and the Jonestown mass suicides regarding founding beliefs and the course of events that led to mass deaths.

Do these observations indicate any further insights or possible areas of prevention?

Key Texts

Reiterman, T. and Jacobs, J. (2008) *Raven: The Untold Story of the Rev. Jim Jones and His People* New York, Penguin.
This book provides a broad account of events and fills out the social context behind the Jonestown deaths.
Singer, M. T. (2003) (Revised edition) *Cults in Our Midst: The Continuing Fight Against Their Hidden Menace* San Francisco, CA, Jossey-Bass.
The book defines cults, considers how they work, and looks at how survivors might be helped to escape and recover.

References

Anderson, D. M. (Chief Lexicographer) (2007). (31st edition). *Dorland's Illustrated Medical Dictionary*. Philadelphia, PA: Saunders Elsevier.

Baronas, D. (2010). *Pilenai and Margiris: History and Legend.* Vilnius: Lithuanian Institute of History.

Bearak, B. (1997, April 28). Eyes on Glory: Pied Pipers of Heaven's Gate. *The New York Times* (Archives). https://www.nytimes.com/1997/04/28/us/eyes-on-glory-pied-pipers-of-heaven-s-gate.html.

Conroy, J. O. (2018, November 17). An Apocalyptic Cult, 900 Dead: Remembering the Jonestown massacre, 40 Years on. *The Guardian.* https://www.theguardian.com/world/2018/nov/17/an-apocalyptic-cult-900-dead-remembering-the-jonestown-massacre-40-years-on.

Contributor. (2015 and 2017). The Jonestown Massacre. *HuffPost* (18 October 2015 and 6 December 2017). https://www.huffpost.com/entry/the-jonestown-massacre_b_8592338.

Eldridge, A. (n.d.). Jonestown: Mass Murder-Suicide, Guyana. *Encyclopaedia Britannica*. https://www.britannica.com/event/Jonestown-massacre.

Fondakowski, L. (2013). *Stories from Jonestown*. Indiana: University of Minnesota Press.

Kumar, P., & Clark, M. (Eds.). (2005). *Clinical Medicine* (6th ed.). London: Elsevier Saunders.

Luther, A. (2018, February 28). The Jonestown Massacre. *The Independent*. www.independent.co.uk/news/world/americas/jonestown-massacre-documentary-40-years-drink-kool-aid-jim-jones-what-happened-mass-suicide-cult-a8232856.html.

Merriam-Webster, accessed December (2019). https://www.merriam-webster.com/dictionary/cult.

Moitt, B. (1996). Slave women and Resistance in the French Caribbean. In D. B. Gaspar (Ed.), *More Than Chattel: Black Women and Slavery in the Americas*. Bloomington and Indianapolis: Indiana University Press.

Moore, R. (2019, March 6). *An Update on the Demographics of Jonestown*. San Diego State University. https://jonestown.sdsu.edu/?page_id=70495.

Reiterman, T., & Jacobs, J. (2008). *Raven: The Untold Story of the Rev. Jim Jones and His People*. New York: Penguin.

Sakellariou, M. V. (1997). *Epirus: 4000 Years of Greek History and Civilisation*. Athens, Greece: Ekdotike Athenon.

Stiebel, Guy D. (2007). Masada. *Encyclopaedia Judaica* Detroit, Macmillan Reference, 593–599.

United States Holocaust Memorial Museum. (accessed 2019). The Warsaw Ghetto Uprising. *Holocaust Encyclopaedia*. https://encyclopedia.ushmm.org/content/en/article/the-warsaw-ghetto-uprising.

Zennie, M. (2012, March 27). New Age followers still waiting for Aliens to Beam Them Up 15 Years After Heaven's Gate Suicide Cult Left 39 People Dead. *The Daily Mail*. https://www.dailymail.co.uk/news/article-2120869/Heavens-Gate-cult-committed-mass-suicide-15-years-ago.html.

8

Capital Punishment by Poisoning

Introduction

Among forms of capital punishment have been hanging, guillotine, and the electric chair while methods involving poison include the gas chamber and lethal injection. Gas chambers typically use hydrogen cyanide while lethal injection comprises a cocktail of various drugs each having different effects. Execution by gas chamber and by lethal injection follow certain procedures. Individual cases of people who have been executed illustrate these and the course of events leading to execution. Situational crime prevention (SCP) can help us to examine strategies to reduce the incidence of capital punishment. This requires focusing not on the condemned person's crime but on the progress of the execution. I examine the means, motive, opportunity, location, and perpetrator–victim relationships with reference to execution by poisoning to highlight the particular circumstances of state-sanctioned capital punishment.

© The Author(s) 2020
M. Farrell, *Criminology of Poisoning Contexts*,
https://doi.org/10.1007/978-3-030-40830-5_8

Definitions of Capital Punishment

The term 'capital punishment' is a misnomer. Punishment is usually intended to inflict pain on a transgressor to deter them from repeating offences later. Clearly, the death sentence ends any possibility of the offender learning from the experience—the deterrence aspect is aimed at others wishing to avoid the same end.

In general definitions, the death penalty is described as 'killing people as punishment for serious crimes' (Merriam-Webster 2019). Similarly, it is punishment involving, 'the legal killing of a person who has committed a serious crime such as murder' (Collins 2019). In the United States, for example, the death penalty can be prescribed by Congress or a state legislature for capital crimes including murder.

History of Capital Punishment

The Code of Hammurabi, a system of law from ancient Mesopotamia (1750s B.C.), Hittite Laws (1650 BC and earlier), and the Roman Law of the Twelve Tablets all included provision for the death penalty.

Drawing and quartering was ordained in 1283 in England for treason. In its full form, the traitor was tied to a horse and dragged to the gallows (drawn). The victim was then hanged, although typically not to death and disembowelled alive, the entrails being burned before him. The offender was then beheaded and cut or pulled into parts (quartered). Sometimes the prisoner was dragged on a sledge possibly to ease suffering, or equally likely, to ensure the victim's live arrival before the gallows (Editors Encyclopaedia Britannica 2019a).

Burning at the stake had ancient origins and was used more recently in Europe and North America. It involved securing the offender to a wooden stake and igniting surrounding kindling. Among well-known victims were Joan of Arc, who was burned as a heretic in 1431 in France; and Bishops Latimer and Ridley burned at Oxford, England, in 1555. To shorten the victim's suffering, a container of gunpowder might be attached to the offender that would explode in the flames killing them instantly (Abbot 2019).

Decapitation was carried out using an axe brought down on a block on which the offender bared their neck. If a sword was used, the victim knelt, and the blade was swung sideways (using a block with a concave hollow would prevent the straight blade cutting through the neck). The guillotine is best known for its introduction in France in 1792. Two upright posts held by a cross beam were grooved to facilitate the smooth descent of a weighted blade onto the neck of an offender lying prone beneath it. Among well-known victims were King Louis XVI and Marie Antoinette during the French Revolution (Editors Encyclopaedia Britannica 2019b).

If any redemptive theme can be glimpsed in these draconian practices, it is occasional attempts to mitigate suffering and speed up death.

Contemporary Methods of Capital Punishment

Modern-day types of capital punishment include hanging, shooting by firing squad, shooting by other means, beheading, electrocution, gas chamber, and lethal injection (Cornell Law School, June 2012).

Hanging is the commonest method of capital punishment. Among countries using it are Afghanistan, Bangladesh, Botswana, India, Iran, Iraq, Japan, Kuwait, Malaysia, Nigeria, the Palestinian Authority in Gaza, South Sudan, and Sudan. Iran carries out many of the executions by hanging (369 people in 2013) (Zahriyeh 2014). Hanging using a 'short drop' could be protracted where the prisoner was suspended by a noose and died by strangulation. Where the drop was too long, the prisoner could be decapitated. In the 1870s, William Marwood refined the 'long drop' aiming to ensure a quick end as the offender died of asphyxia while unconscious. Relatedly, in 1888 the UK Home office published a table showing the length of rope required to lead to quick execution considering the prisoner's weight and build. In September 2017, Iranian authorities publicly hanged Esmail Jafarzadeh for raping and murdering a seven-year-old girl (Moore 2017).

Firing squad is used in China, Indonesia, North Korea, Saudi Arabia, Somalia, Taiwan, United Arab Emirates, and Yemen. Typically, the prisoner is restrained, before several armed executioners open fire. The offender may be standing or, if there is reason, for example a prior leg injury, the prisoner may be secured to a chair. If necessary, the commander shoots a final bullet into the person's head. On 18 January 2015, Nigerian Daniel Enemuo was executed by firing squad in Indonesia for drug offenses (Banjo 2015). Shooting other than by firing squad involves a single firearm shot to the prisoner's head.

Stoning has been used in Afghanistan, Nigeria, Iran, Pakistan, Sudan, Saudi Arabia, and the United Arab Emirates. In preparation men are buried up to the waist and women up to the neck. On 5 July 2007, in the Qazvin Province of Iran, Jaffar Kiani was stoned to death for adultery (BBC News, 10 July 2007).

Beheading is officially used as a capital punishment only in Saudi Arabia and is carried out publicly using a sword. In January 2013, a domestic worker Rizana Nafeek from Sri Lanka was beheaded for smothering to death a baby in her care (BBC News 9 January 2013).

Electrocution has been used in the United States. The condemned person is strapped to a specially constructed padded chair and electrocuted through electrodes fitted to the head and legs. A brine-soaked sponge is strapped to the prisoner's calf and scalp to hasten death by speeding up the current's passage through the body. Robert Gleason Jr. was electrocuted in Virginia on 16 January 2013 for murdering two prison inmates (Zahriyeh 2014).

Other currently used types of capital punishment are the gas chamber and lethal injection, considered later. The action of the poisons used in capital punishment are described in the earlier chapter, 'Poisoning and its contexts'.

Capital Punishment: Arguments for and Against

Capital punishment is used for crimes considered very serious in the society in which they are applied. These include in different jurisdictions, adultery, treason, and murder. In this section I concentrate on capital punishment for murder, which is universally considered a most serious crime. Positions for and against capital punishment can be variously classified, for example, moral, utilitarian, and practical arguments (Hood 2019). In these debates, different evidence and different interpretations of evidence are used to support each view. Here I mention a few issues.

Moral Positions

Moral positions on the death penalty sometimes distinguish murder from other serious crimes. Proponents maintain that if murder is committed, the perpetrator has in taking life given up any claim to life themselves. At the same time, it is justified for state representatives to take the life of the murderer as retribution on behalf of outraged relatives of the victim and other members of society. Opponents put the view that if the state legally sanctions and carries out the death penalty for murder, it condones killing, the very phenomenon that it claims to abhor. Therefore, the moral message is inconsistent and confused.

A further argument is that there is an essential right to life (whatever the perpetrator has done) and that the state by taking an offender's life is violating this professed right. A counterargument is that the right to life is not inviolable but can be forfeited in certain circumstances, and that having committed murder is an example. Relatedly, it may be proposed that capital punishment is inherently inhuman and degrading.

Religious Injunctions

While views on capital punishment can draw on moral positions, they can also refer to articles of faith believed to come from God. Foundational texts of religious faiths including Judaism and Christianity prescribe death for crimes including murder ('an eye for an eye'). In the modern day, such strictures are not always accepted. Religious authorities and believers may differ about their interpretations and on the position that they take towards capital punishment.

Deterrence

A key area of debate is the extent to which capital punishment acts as a deterrent. Proponents claim that the ultimate penalty is a unique deterrent to murder and other very serious crimes, compared with other punishments. Opponents maintain that the death penalty is no more or less of a deterrent than other sanctions such as long terms of imprisonment.

Added to these debates are occasions when an offender imprisoned for a very serious crime is eventually released and goes on to commit a further serious offence such as murder. It may then be claimed that, if the perpetrator had remained in prison, they would have not been able to offend again. Opposed to this is the position that while in prison more could be done to rehabilitate offenders making it less likely that they will offend again on release.

Systemic Injustices

It is debated whether capital punishment can be just or whether there are systemic problems in any system that preclude justice. Proponents claim that laws and related procedures can be formed to ensure that the death penalty reflects a just response to grave wrongdoing.

Opponents may argue that social and cultural features may prevent the 'fair' application of the death penalty. In some countries it may be argued that poor people or individuals of a minority ethnic background (in that culture) do not have the same access to the best legal help compared with rich people or those from a majority ethnic background. Therefore, there is an increased likelihood that some individuals will be sentenced in part in relation to their material wealth and their ethnicity. Evidence may be provided to support this claim. In response the legislature may take steps to try to ensure more equitable legal representation.

Another concern is that in countries where there is a white majority, and black people are in a minority, and where there is racial prejudice, there may be inequities in the allocation of capital punishment. In capital cases, it may be claimed, mainly white juries will convict disproportionally more black defendants than white defendants where there is no apparent justification. One response to this concern is jury selection agreeable to both prosecution and defence lawyers.

It is also pointed out that even in the best judicial system there will inevitably be mistakes, leading to innocent people being executed. One response is to try to continually improve the system of justice so that it keeps public confidence.

Objections to Certain Types of Capital Punishment

It may be argued that certain methods of carrying out the death penalty make death too protracted or cause unnecessary suffering. This position can be used to oppose a certain form of execution such as electrocution because it is believed to cause unnecessary pain and suffering but may leave the door open to the use of other methods which are perceived to be more humane. More commonly, it is argued that each method is inhumane, perhaps for different reasons. This arises where lawyers appeal against the only method used by a legislature on the grounds that it is inhumane. Effectively, this becomes an argument for abolishing capital punishment in that legislation.

Situational Crime Prevention

SCP is fully described in the chapter 'Theory and Poison Contexts'. Briefly, five general strategies are each associated with five opportunity-reducing techniques. Regarding the strategy **increase the effort** of perpetrators are the strategies 'target harden', 'control access to facilities', 'screen exits', 'deflect offenders', and 'control tools/weapons'. **Increase the risks** concerns 'extend guardianship', 'assist natural surveillance', 'reduce anonymity', 'utilise place managers', and 'strengthen formal surveillance'. For **reduce rewards** to the perpetrator, the techniques are 'conceal targets', 'remove targets', 'identify property', 'disrupt markets', and 'deny benefits'. Regarding **reduce provocations**, techniques comprise 'reduce frustrations and stress', 'avoid disputes', 'reduce emotional arousal', 'neutralise peer pressure', and 'discourage imitation'. **Remove excuses** concerns 'set rules', 'post instructions', 'alert conscience', 'assist compliance', and 'control drugs and alcohol'.

Gas chamber: Procedures, Prevalence, and a Case

Procedures for Gas Chamber Execution

A gas chamber used for capital punishment is a sealed room in which two chemicals are brought together to produce hydrogen cyanide gas which kills the prisoner located in the room. The chamber is fitted with a chair behind which (out of the chair occupant's line of sight) are windows for witnesses to view the execution. Underneath the chair is a compartment containing potassium cyanide pellets. In an adjacent room are vessels of sulphuric acid connected by tubes to a holding compartment of the chair.

The prisoner is brought in by staff, strapped to the chair, and fitted with a chest stethoscope to monitor heart rate. Once staff have exited, the door is sealed. From the room containing the sulphuric acid, the executioner releases an amount through the tubes and into the chair's holding compartment. Next, the executioner operates a lever allowing the acid and cyanide pellets to mix, producing hydrogen cyanide gas.

Usually, the prisoner dies within several minutes and this is confirmed by the cessation of heartbeat indicated by the stethoscope soundings. Gas is then extracted from the chamber and the space is neutralised with anhydrous ammonia. Staff wearing oxygen masks then enter the chamber and remove the body for a physician to examine.

Prevalence of Gas Chamber Execution

In the United States, the numbers of individuals executed by gas chamber declined from the 1920s, when the method was introduced, to 1999, when the last execution took place in Arizona. Currently, only four states allow for execution by gas chamber and all offer lethal injection as an alternative. An advance count of executions in 2017 showed that from 1 January to 31 December 2017, 23 prisoners were executed, none by gas chamber (Davis and Snell, April 2018, p. 8).

Robert Alton Harris—Towards Execution

Robert Alton Harris was executed by gas chamber in 1978 for murder. Steps taken to delay or annul his execution illustrate some of the arguments against the death penalty.

Born in Fort Bragg, North Carolina, Robert Alton Harris was the fifth of nine children. His father Kenneth was a decorated sergeant of the US Army. Both father and mother Evelyn had alcohol problems. It is reported that Robert was physically abused by his father who believed that Robert was not his child. Following Kenneth's army discharge, the family moved to Visalia, California, in 1962. Jailed in both 1963 and 1964 for sexually abusing his daughters, Kenneth Harris left his family members to a migrant existence wandering the San Joaquin Valley.

At age 13, having stolen a car, Robert spent four months in a juvenile detention centre where it is reported that he was repeatedly raped. In 1967, Evelyn abandoned 14-year-old Robert in Sacramento and the boy made his way to Oklahoma to stay with his brother and sister.

Later he was arrested in Florida for car stealing and spent three years in juvenile detention. At age 19, he was sent to California. In June 1973, Harris married. Two years later, he beat his brother's roommate to death without provocation. Convicted of voluntary manslaughter Harris was imprisoned during which time his wife filed for divorce. Harris was paroled in January 1978, aged 25.

Soon afterwards, Robert and his brother Daniel, 18, planned a bank robbery. On July 2, Daniel stole two guns, and the pair drove to San

Diego and spent two days preparing near Miramar Lake. On July 5, the brothers came across John Mayeski and Michael Baker, both 16, sitting in a car in a parking lot in Mira Mesa prior to a day's fishing trip. Robert Harris commandeered Mayeski's car and ordered him to drive to Miramar Lake saying they would use the vehicle to rob a bank. Daniel Harris followed in another vehicle. At the Lake, the Harris brothers shot the boys dead before returning to Robert's Mira Mesa home. An hour later, the Harris brothers robbed the local bank of $2000 but were arrested shortly after. One of the arresting officers, Steven Baker, was the unsuspecting father of victim Michael Baker.

On 6 March 1979, Robert Harris was convicted in the San Diego Court of murder and kidnapping and sentenced to death. Daniel was imprisoned for kidnapping. An appeal for clemency was rejected by California governor Wilson, who acknowledged Harris's abusive childhood but said this did not excuse the crimes. In 1990, an appeal was lodged that Harris had childhood brain damage which affected his judgement during his offences. In 1992, a further appeal challenged the constitutionality of the gas chamber as a method of execution. In April 1992, at San Quentin State Prison gas chamber, the execution order was given at 6:07 am and Harris died at 6:21 am (Clarke County Prosecuting Attorney's Office, various dates).

Robert Alton Harris Execution—Analysis

We turn now to an interpretation of capital punishment informed by SCP, particularly prevention. **Increasing the effort** of perpetrators includes *hardening targets* which, applied to a condemned person, implies appealing against the penalty. With Harris, repeated appeals delaying execution included a request for clemency, a claim that brain damage had affected Harris's judgement during his crime, and the argument that using the gas chamber was unconstitutional. *Controlling tools/weapons* involves attempts to disrupt the supply of poisons for executions or arguing for their prohibition. Concerning Harris, Ninth Court judges maintained that the use of the gas chamber was unconstitutional.

Increasing the risks to the perpetrator through enhancing *natural* and *formal surveillance* relates to publicising witness information on death penalty procedures. Information about Harris's execution, while not preventive for him, might be later cited to illustrate that gas chamber death may be prolonged and may cause unnecessary suffering. *Reducing anonymity* can relate to publicising the participation of those involved in the execution exposing them to possible public opposition. This appears not to have been done in the Harris execution, except for making known its duration.

Reducing rewards to the perpetrator through *concealing* and *removing targets* relates to the earlier issue of hardening targets through the appeals process, for example the request for clemency based on Harris's brutal childhood experiences. To *deny benefits* can be to argue against the death penalty, for example maintaining that mistakes can lead to an innocent person being executed. Harris's representatives did not claim his innocence presumably because of the strong evidence against him.

Reducing provocations normally implies that the perpetrator is provoked to commit a crime. Therefore, preventive approaches directed at the potential perpetrator are 'reducing frustrations and stress', 'avoiding disputes', 'reducing emotional arousal', 'neutralising peer pressure', and 'discouraging imitation'. However, with capital punishment the condemned person is not executed because the executioner suddenly feels frustrated and stressed. Neither is the executioner, in dispute with the prisoner, emotionally aroused to kill, driven by peer pressure, or intent on imitating someone else. The executioner does a job required by the state at a set time and in an agreed place. Consequently, reducing provocations does not apply to state executions and is not discussed further in the examples considered later.

Concerning **removing excuses**, 'set rules' applied to a legal claim that the 'rules' of the constitution were being violated by executing Harris by gas chamber.

Lethal Injection: Procedures, Prevalence, and Cases

Procedures for Lethal Injection Execution

Death penalty by lethal injection has typically used a combination of drugs delivered in sequence. These are sodium thiopental or pentobarbital (a short-acting barbiturate anaesthetic causing unconsciousness and depressing respiration), pancuronium bromide (a total muscle relaxant causing paralysis of muscles including the diaphragm and other respiratory muscles), and potassium chloride (a substance inducing cardiac arrest).

In the United States, the condemned person is strapped to a gurney and into their arm is inserted an intravenous canula (a tube allowing fluid to be introduced into or removed from the body). This is connected to a line that leads into an adjacent room. A backup IV line is inserted into the other arm. To ensure that the lines are flowing correctly, a saline drip is started. A heart monitor is connected to the prisoner. Next, a curtain previously concealing the execution chamber is drawn back to allow witnesses to view the procedure and for the prisoner, if desired, to make a statement. When the execution begins, the drugs are introduced in sequence. Death is pronounced when the monitor shows that cardiac action has stopped. This is usually about seven minutes after the procedure starts unless there are delays such as difficulty finding a suitable vein.

Some states have switched to a single-drug protocol for lethal injection using sodium thiopental, Ohio being the first in 2009. Responding to groups opposing capital punishment, manufacturers of sodium thiopental and pentobarbital stopped supplying US prisons and ordered their resellers to do likewise.

Prevalence of Lethal Injection Execution

In the United States, 23 male prisoners were executed between January and December 2017, in eight states, as follows: Texas (7 prisoners), Arkansas (4), Alabama (3), Florida (3), Ohio (2), Virginia (2), Missouri (1), and Georgia (1). All these executions were by lethal injection. No women were executed (Davis and Snell, April 2018, p. 8).

Danny Bible: Towards Execution

In May 1979, the body of 20-year-old Inez Deaton was found in a field in Harris County. She had been raped and stabbed with an ice pick. Her murder went unsolved until 1998. Then, Danny Bible was arrested in Louisiana in another rape case and confessed to that rape as well as Deaton's murder. Bible told police that Deaton, a friend of his cousin, walked into his uncle's house where he was staying. Bible raped her, stabbed her to death, and dumped her body. He fled Texas when the corpse was discovered shortly after the murder. Bible also confessed to the murders in 1983 of his former sister-in-law, her baby, and her roommate. He had already served a prison sentence for one of these killings but was paroled. Sentenced to death for Deaton's murder, Bible made several appeals (McCullough 2018).

One appeal concerned Bible's illness and supposed failed veins. Attorneys claimed that lethal injection could cause a botched or aborted execution because of Bible's heart and lung conditions and Parkinson's Disease. Bible would likely choke laying on his back on the gurney. His veins were too weak for the IVs; indeed, other execution attempts on sick inmates had failed because officials could not locate a suitable vein. They proposed considering the use of a firing squad or nitrogen gas. The state responded referencing the severity of Bible's crimes and stating that his claims of an inhumane and painful execution were speculative. Also, the failed vein claim was hypothetical, and the alternatives also posed a risk. The US Supreme Court rejected Bible's appeal.

Bible also argued that he should be granted a new punishment trial. This takes place after a person has been found guilty of capital murder. In Texas, to sentence someone to death (rather than life in prison) jurors must unanimously agree that the prisoner is a future danger. In 2003, having been sentenced to death, Bible was being transferred from the county jail to death row when his prison van crashed killing the driver and leaving Bible unable to walk without assistance. In the Texas Court of Criminal Appeals, it was argued that because of this accident and the associated disability, jurors may not deem Bible a future danger. This appeal was also rejected. In June 2018, Bible was executed by lethal injection.

Danny Bible Execution: Analysis

Increasing the effort of perpetrators through *hardening the target* (the condemned person) related to Bible's appeals. These concerned a request for clemency, and reference to his illnesses, possible failed veins, and his post-punishment trial injury. *Controlling tools/weapons* relates to attempts to hinder the supply of execution poisons or arguing for their prohibition. Bible's representatives claimed that the drugs, although available, should be prohibited because of the risk of a botched or aborted execution.

Increasing the risks to perpetrators includes enhancing *natural* and *formal surveillance*. Both apply to publicising details of death penalty procedures on other prisoners. Bible's lawyers cited earlier instances where executions had been cancelled. Lawyers seemingly did not try to *reduce anonymity* (and exert public pressure) by publicising the participation of those involved in the execution.

With reference to **reducing rewards** to perpetrators, *concealing* and *removing targets* relate to Bible's appeal requesting clemency, but the parole board rejected this. *Denying benefits* by arguing that mistakes can lead to an innocent person being executed was not feasible because Bible had confessed.

Removing excuses with reference to *setting rules* involved a legal argument that the 'rules' of the lethal injection protocol could not likely be followed because of Bible's illnesses and possible failed veins.

Ronald Phillips: Towards Execution

Ronald Phillips (1973–2017) was executed in Ohio by lethal injection for the rape and murder of three-year-old Sheila Evans. The child was the daughter of Phillips' girlfriend Fae Evans, who with Ronald Phillips was implicated in prolonged physical and sexual abuse of the child. (Fae Evans was sentenced to 30 years imprisonment for involuntary manslaughter and died in prison.) Born in Akron Ohio, Phillips was the fifth of seven children. It is reported that as a child he was physically and sexually abused by his father.

Phillips was sentenced in 1993. Between 2013 and 2017, he was scheduled for execution nine times. A November 2013 date was halted when Phillips asked permission to donate non-vital organs prior to his execution. This was denied on the grounds that he would not have time to recover before his rescheduled execution date of July 2014.

Phillips (and several other prisoners) sought stays of execution on the grounds of the constitutionality of Ohio's lethal injection protocol and the question of whether Ohio were able to procure the requisite drugs. A preliminary injunction was granted to the prisoners in January 2017, but the Court of Appeals for the Sixth Circuit ruled in favour of the State of Ohio. After further unsuccessful appeals, Phillips was executed on 26 July 2017.

Ronald Phillips Execution: Analysis

Increasing the effort of perpetrators through *hardening targets* relates to Phillips's appeals to delay his execution including a request to be allowed to donate organs. Regarding *controlling tools/weapons*, Phillips' lawyers argued that the execution drugs may not have been available, and that aspects of the protocol were unconstitutional.

With reference to **increasing the risks** to the perpetrator, *reducing anonymity* can relate to challenging and publicising the execution protocol to exert public pressure. Phillips' lawyers accordingly challenged the constitutionality of the procedure and questioned the availability of the requisite drugs.

Reducing rewards to the perpetrator includes *concealing* and *removing targets* in relation to which Phillips' lawyers questioned the constitutionality of the execution. *Denying benefits* can involve arguing that mistakes can lead to an innocent person being executed, but evidence of Phillips' guilt was clear.

Concerning **removing excuses**, *setting rules* involved Phillips' lawyers arguing that the 'rules' of the lethal injection protocol were unconstitutional.

Situational Crime Prevention: Overview

SCP and Capital Punishment

Normally, in applying SCP the perpetrator commits or attempts a crime, and efforts are made to identify aspects of the situation that can be influenced to deter the offense. With the death penalty, the focus is not on the crime committed by the condemned person, but on the act of execution as a state-sanctioned punishment. Also, viewing the execution as the homicide to be prevented, the situation in which the condemned person is executed hardly allows direct intervention. Any preventive actions must occur much earlier so that prevention focuses on averting a sequence of actions leading to the end point of state execution.

Increase the Effort

With a condemned person, *hardening a target* implies appealing the sentence hoping for one successful appeal, or for new exonerating evidence. Harris's appeals concerned clemency, the prisoner's brain damage, and the unconstitutionality of the gas chamber. Bible's grounds were clemency, his illnesses and possible failed veins, and his incapacitating injury. Phillips argued for permission to donate organs, and that the lethal injection protocol was unconstitutional.

Controlling tools/weapons can concern attempts to disrupt or hinder the supply of poisons used for executions, or arguments for the prohibition of the use of poisons. Harris claimed that the gas chamber was unconstitutional. Bible argued that lethal injection drugs should be prohibited as they risked a botched or aborted execution. Phillips questioned the availability of the necessary drugs and maintained that the lethal injection protocol was unconstitutional.

Increase the Risks

Enhancing *natural* and *formal surveillance* can raise public awareness of death penalty procedures. Sources can be execution witnesses such as prison staff (guards, chaplain, governor), journalists, and those directly involved in preparing the condemned person and carrying out the execution. The expectation is that where humanising details are publicised, or even botched procedures, public appetite for the death penalty might diminish. The duration of Harris's execution was made public, showing it as protracted and possibly causing unnecessary suffering. With Bible, examples of earlier instances of cancelled executions were cited.

Reducing anonymity can include publicising and exposing to possible public pressure those implicated in the execution, including manufacturers and suppliers of drugs to US prisons. Accordingly, Phillips's lawyers challenged the constitutionality of lethal injection procedures and questioned whether the requisite drugs would be available.

Reduce Rewards

Concealing and *removing targets* concerns appeals delaying the execution and has the same implications as hardening targets already discussed.

To *deny benefits* can be to argue against the death penalty yielding benefits. Proponents of capital punishment guarantees that the offender will never offend again. Opponents may point out that if later exonerating information came to light, it is too late to make reparations if the prisoner has been executed. The argument about future exonerating information could not be made regarding Harris or Phillips because the evidence was unequivocal, while Bible confessed to the murder for which he was executed.

Remove Excuses

Removing excuses relates to claims that proponents use excuses to continue the practice of capital punishment. Attempts to remove perceived excuses constitute another way of arguing against capital punishment. For example, death penalty proponents may point out that most of the world's population live in jurisdictions that support the death sentence, suggesting that the majority view prevails. Opponents may note that most countries do not have the death penalty, highlighting that most legislatures oppose it.

With reference to *setting rules* it was argued that constitutional 'rules' were violated by using the gas chamber (Harris) and lethal injection (Phillips) and that a particular execution would likely not comply with lethal injection protocols (Bible).

Means, Motive, Opportunity, Location, and Perpetrator–Victim Relationship

Discussing means, motive, opportunity, location, and perpetrator–victim relationship usually focuses on the criminal perpetrator and a range of possible offences including homicide. Here, I look at how these features might apply to state endorsed killing. Each feature therefore takes on a different complexion highlighting differences between criminal and legally sanctioned homicide.

Means

The effectiveness and relative humaneness of the means or methods of capital punishment have long been debated. Sir Norwood East prepared a memorandum for a Royal Commission in the United Kingdom (The Royal Commission 1949–1952, p. 511). He considered hanging the 'best method', although electrocution was 'no doubt painless'. Shooting, he thought 'noisy' and 'unnecessarily complex' while beheading was likely to 'affront public opinion'. Regarding execution by poison, East distinguished between subcutaneous and intravenous injections, poison administered in food or drink, and poison gas. He concluded, 'There is an element of secrecy in the use of poison which is repugnant to most people' (Ibid.). While some of East's views may seem naïve today, opinions on the relative merits and demerits of methods of execution are still debated.

An argument sometimes used in support of hanging is the speed with which it can be done in a prison setting. With Albert Pierrepoint, the UK hangman, the time between his entering the condemned cell and the death of the prisoner was typically a few seconds (Pierrepoint 1991

[1974], p. 176 and passim). East's view about the secrecy of poison derives from its usually secretive criminal use, but has not influenced the modern use of lethal injection in the United States.

Opponents of lethal injection in the United States have claimed that it presents an unacceptable risk of suffering. Some states, it is argued, used a drug combination making it impossible to know whether a prisoner is conscious or not when receiving the fatal dose of potassium chloride. This drug causes pain if the prisoner is not anaesthetised. Further procedural problems can be drugs administered improperly and a purported lack of clinical evidence that the drugs are safe and effective. In the cases of *Baze v Rees* (2008), the US Supreme Court rejected these arguments. They determined that a prisoner must be able to show that the state's lethal injection protocol 'creates a demonstrated risk of severe pain'. This risk must be substantial when compared to other alternative methods (Cornell Law School, 22 June 2012).

Motive

Motive does not apply to a state executioner in the usual sense that it applies to a criminal homicide. Normally, a perpetrator commits a crime for some advantage such as monetary gain or escape from an unwanted relationship. Homicide may occur in relation to a sexual or aggressive interaction. An executioner acts towards a prisoner not out of personal motives such as these but as an agent of the state. There may be secondary motives such as wanting to do an efficient job as is evident in Pierrepoint's autobiography (Pierrepoint 1991 [1974], passim). However, this does not constitute a direct motive for killing.

Opportunity

Opportunity too has a different emphasis. Unlike a criminal perpetrator, an executioner does not wait for and seize an opportunity to kill but is guided by the legal process which can last many years. Neither is the opportunity fleeting or random. A date and time are set in advance, and the killing is carried out according to formal guidelines or protocols.

Location

Normally, the location of an execution is a prison where the condemned person is held. Within the prison, the exact location is predetermined and shaped according to the type of execution. With the gas chamber and lethal injection, a dedicated space is set aside and designed according to the requirements of the death penalty. Usually, the area is near the condemned cell. The chamber in which the prisoner dies and the room from which the poison is released are separated. In its design, the execution chamber may enable witnesses to see the death and allow the prisoner to deliver a final statement

Perpetrator–Victim Relationship

The perpetrator–victim relationship in criminal homicide can indicate certain demographic patterns. For male on male general homicides, often the participants are acquaintances (30%) or strangers (20%), after which come friends (10%) and family members (7%) (Brookman 2005, p. 122). With femicide, over a half of women victims are killed by their current or former boyfriend, husband, or lover and fewer than 10% are killed by a stranger (Ibid. p. 141). When women kill, victims tend to be intimate partners, ex-partners, or family members (their children) (Ibid. pp. 162–163).

Such demographic patterns are not pertinent to executions. Capital punishment involves not a personal relationship but a formal role. The executioner carries out a requirement of a legal system. Prisoners' gender, social background, race, and age may reflect social forces and norms within a society. A greater or smaller proportion of some racial groups may face execution than is expected according to their preponderance in the wider society. Also, there is a lower age limit in many countries below which a person (child) is not considered culpable for a crime and would not face execution. However, the executioner does not select those to be killed on any such criteria but carries out the task as a legal duty.

Conclusion

Situational Crime Prevention

Behavioural and situational levers contributing to SCP can be interpreted as strategies to prevent execution, and how they are circumvented. *Target hardening* relating to a condemned person, implies legal appeals. Lawyers hope these will create time for a successful appeal or new exonerating evidence to emerge. *Controlling tools/weapons* concerns attempts to disrupt or hinder the supply of execution poisons and arguments for their prohibition.

Enhancing *natural* and *formal surveillance* can draw public attention to details of death penalty procedures, citing witnesses to the execution. Publicising humanising or harrowing details aims to turn public opinion against the death penalty. *Reducing anonymity* can expose participants in the execution to possible public opposition. Lawyers may challenge the constitutionality of the lethal injection procedure and question if (under public pressure) companies will supply the drugs.

Concealing and *removing targets* involves delaying execution, allowing time for a successful appeal or for new exculpatory evidence. To *deny benefits* involves arguing that the death penalty offers no benefits. Claimed benefit are that an executed person can never offend again, and the death penalty is a deterrent. Against this it is claimed that exculpatory evidence might emerge post-execution too late for the state to make reparations and that deterrence is non-existent or limited.

Removing excuses applies to claims that proponents are using spurious reasons to continue capital punishment. Proponents and opponents of the death penalty are likely to choose different evidence and interpretations to support their views. *Setting rules* applies to 'rules' like those implied in the US constitution and how they might be interpreted.

Means, Motive, Opportunity, Location, and Perpetrator–Victim Relationship

Opponents of lethal injection claim that it presents an unacceptable risk of suffering. Some states of the United States, it was argued, used a drug combination making it impossible to know whether a prisoner experienced pain. There were disputes about whether the drugs were safe, effective, or administered properly. However, the US Supreme Court tended not to accept these arguments (Cornell Law School, 22 June 2012).

Motive does not apply to an executioner as it does to a perpetrator of criminal homicide. When a perpetrator commits murder, the motive is normally advantageous, for example financial gain, or it may involve sexual or aggressive interaction. In contrast, an executioner acts towards a prisoner as an agent of the state system of punishment for crime.

An executioner does not, as do criminal perpetrators, await and seize an *opportunity* to kill but is guided by the legal process, is bound by an agreed date and time, and follows protocols.

Normally, the *location* of an execution is a prison holding the condemned person. With the gas chamber and lethal injection, the exact locations, adjoining rooms, and other aspects of design are formalised.

In a criminal homicide, *perpetrator–victim relationships* show different demographic patterns (Brookman 2005, pp. 122, 141). These are not pertinent to execution because it involves a legal, not a personal, relationship. Prisoner demographics may reflect social forces and norms. However, the executioner does not select those to be killed on any such criteria but acts according to a legal duty.

Suggested Activities

With reference to capital punishment by lethal injection, which arguments for and against it are the most sustainable? What are likely to be the best grounds for appeal against death penalty by lethal injection?

Regarding countries currently using methods of execution that some other jurisdictions might consider barbaric, it may be argued that this acts as a surer deterrent to others keeping society safer. Try to rigorously present legal, moral, and societal arguments on either side of this position with statistical and other evidence, if available.

Key Texts

Bohm, R. M. and Lee, G. (Eds.) (2019) *The Routledge Handbook on Capital Punishment* London and New York, Routledge.
Sections of the book consider capital punishment in relation to history, opinion. and culture; rationales and religious views; constitutional issues; administration of the death penalty; and consequences of the death penalty.
Hood, R, and Hoyle, C. (5th Edition) (2015) *The Death Penalty: A Worldwide Perspective* Oxford, Oxford University Press.
Chapters of particular interest include 'The Scope of Capital Punishment in Law and Practice', 'The Death Penalty in Practice: The Process of Execution and the Death Row Experience', and 'Protecting the Accused and Ensuring Due Process'.
Steiker, C. S. and Steiker, J. M. (2015) *Courting Death: The Supreme Court and Capital Punishment* Cambridge, Massachusetts, The Belknap Press of Harvard University Press.
The book examines the history of the top-down judicial regulation of capital punishment under the US constitution and its contemporary consequences.

References

Abbot, G. (2019). Burning at the Stake – Capital Punishment. *Encyclopaedia Britannica*. https://www.britannica.com/topic/burning-at-the-stake.
Banjo, T. (2015, January 18). Nigerian Drug Convict, 5 Others Executed by Firing Squad. *Nigerian Monitor*. http://www.nigerianmonitor.com/photos-nigerian-drug-convict-5-others-executed-by-firing-squad-in-indonesia/.
Baze v. Rees. (2008). *Baze v. Rees* 553 U.S. 35.
BBC News. (2007, July 10). Iran Adulterer Stoned to Death. http://news.bbc.co.uk/1/hi/world/middle_east/6288156.stm.
BBC News. (2013, January 9). Sri Lankan Maid Rizana Nafeek beheaded in Saudi Arabia. www.bbc.co.uk/news/world-asia-20959228.
Brookman, F. (2005). *Understanding Homicide*. London and Los Angeles: Sage.

Collins. (2019). Capital Punishment. *Collins Dictionary*. https://www.collins-dictionary.com/dictionary/english/capital-punishment.

Cornell Law School. (2012, June). *Methods of Execution* Cornell Centre on the Death Penalty Worldwide http://www.deathpenaltyworldwide.org/methods-of-execution.cfm.

Davis, E., & Snell, T. L. (2018, April). *Capital Punishment 2016* (NCJ 251430) U.S. Department of Justice Office of Justice Programs Bureau of Justice Statistics.

Department of Justice Office of Justice Programs Bureau of Justice Statistics.

Editors Encyclopaedia Britannica. (2019a). Drawing and Quartering – Capital Punishment. *Encyclopaedia Britannica*. https://www.britannica.com/topic/drawing-and-quartering.

Editors Encyclopaedia Britannica. (2019b). Guillotine – Execution Device. *Encyclopaedia Britannica*. https://www.britannica.com/topic/guillotine.

Hood, R. (2019). Arguments for and Against Capital Punishment. *Encyclopaedia Britannica*. https://www.britannica.com/topic/capital-punishment/Arguments-for-and-against-capital-punishment.

Clarke County Prosecuting Attorney's Office (various dates) http://www.clark-prosecutor.org/html/death/US/harris169.htm.

McCullough, J. (2018, June 27). Danny Bible Executed for a 1979 Rape and Murder, Despite Claims That He Was Too Sick for Lethal Injection. *Texas Tribune*. https://www.texastribune.org/2018/06/27/danny-bible-faces-execution-1979-texas-rape-and-murder-he-says-hes-too/.

Merriam-Webster. (2019). Capital Punishment. *Merriam-Webster Dictionary*. https://www.merriam-webster.com/dictionary/capital%20punishment.

Moore, J. (2017, September 20). Iran Publicly Hangs Man for Rape, Murder of Seven-Year-Old Girl' *Newsweek*.

Pierrepoint, A. (1991 [1974]). *Executioner: Pierrepoint – The Amazing Autobiography of the World's Most Famous Executioner*. London: Hodder and Stoughton/Coronet Books.

The Royal Commission. (1949–1952). *Minutes of Evidence Taken Before the Royal Commission on Capital Punishment*. London: Her Majesty's Stationary Office.

Zahriyeh, E. (2014, April 30). Execution Methods Around the World. *Aljazeera America*. http://america.aljazeera.com/articles/2014/4/30/execution-methods.html.

9

Implications of poisoning contexts

Introduction

Here, I consider the contexts of healthcare serial poisoning, assassination, terrorism, warfare, mass suicide, and capital punishment. For each I summarise means, motive, opportunity, location, and perpetrator–victim demographics and relationships and at 'evasion' by the perpetrator and at the 'response' of others.

Means, Motive, Opportunity, Location, and Perpetrator–Victim Relationship Across Different Contexts

Means

Regarding health care serial poisoners, patients are typically poisoned through overdoses of medication. Where this occurs, it may involve an abuse of the duties of specialist nurses and others looking after patients with heart problems, respiratory difficulties, and diabetes. Poisoners may

© The Author(s) 2020
M. Farrell, *Criminology of Poisoning Contexts*,
https://doi.org/10.1007/978-3-030-40830-5_9

take advantage of the trust they enjoy when giving overdoses of the drug used in treatment to create signs and symptoms that can be mistaken for the patient's illness.

In assassination, poisoning's delayed action can allow the killer to escape. Slow-acting poisoning gives no indication to potential witnesses of any attack taking place so that even if traced, witnesses are unlikely to recall anything pertinent. Where poisoning results in a victim's long, painful death, it powerfully deters others such as political dissidents and critics.

In a terrorist attack, the perpetrator can release a poison and unsuspiciously depart in a vehicle or walk safely away. In this manner, poisons enable killing to take place as the perpetrator escapes, leaving victims unaware of the danger.

Chemical weapons are used in warfare because they can cause lingering death, affecting troop morale, and terrorising civilians. Hard-to-detect colourless and odourless poisonous agents make it difficult for victims to take precautions increasing the fear that the poisons generate.

Poison used for cult mass suicide promises speedy death without excessive suffering, and without causing further alarm through bloodshed. Additional means like alcohol may be used to accelerate death or make it less distressing.

Supporters see the use of poisons in capital punishment as a more humane form of execution than some alternatives. In the United States, opponents of lethal injection claimed that it presented an unacceptable risk of suffering. Some states, it was argued, used a drug combination effectively masking whether a prisoner experienced pain when receiving the fatal dose of potassium chloride. Disputes arose about whether the drugs were safe, effective, or administered properly.

Poison is used in these contexts for different reasons and because of its different properties and effects. It can be mistaken for death by natural causes or illness. It can cause slow death rendering an attack unnoticed and allowing a perpetrator to escape. Poison can be left somewhere to have a delayed effect. It can terrorise by causing slow unpleasant death and being difficult to protect against. Poison can be preferred because it allows a less-painful death than some alternatives. In brief, poisoning is used knowingly for its preferred effects.

Motive

Healthcare serial poisoners may seek excitement, self-aggrandisement, and sadistic satisfaction, and may claim (unjustifiably) that they are carrying out mercy killing. More rarely, financial gain, jealousy, and revenge are the drivers (Farrell 2018, pp. 100–107). A poisoner may intervene to rescue patients from the jeopardy that the perpetrator has created or may have the warped notion that they are reducing the health burden on society.

With assassination, the background political motive for poisoning may be to exact revenge, to create a warning to others, or to remove someone who is proving a nuisance to a regime.

Terrorist attacks (including ones using poison) tend to be ideological so target broad groups or random victims rather than specific individuals. Where terrorists despise their host culture, the motive may be to harm 'society' in a wider sense.

In warfare, chemical weapons are used to defeat or weaken opposing forces and to demoralise troops and civilians. In fact, the motives are like those for using other non-chemical weapons in warfare.

Regarding mass suicides, cult leaders may be motivated by guidance from a supposed higher power. They may be initially driven by hopes of social justice, but this may gradually be corrupted by their own paranoia and a desire to control followers. Leaders' suicide may be to escape worldly consequences including crimes. Followers may believe in the cult leaders and their revelations or may more unthinkingly obey the leader's orders. Both leaders and followers may think that they are resisting to malign earthly authorities or gaining entry to a heavenly afterlife.

With capital punishment, motive does not apply to the executioner as it does to a perpetrator of criminal homicide. A criminal may kill for monetary gain or to escape from an unwanted relationship or because of sexual or aggressive impulses. An executioner kills not as a perpetrator driven by such personal and attitudinal motives but as an agent of the state system of punishment for crime.

Opportunity

Opportunity for a healthcare worker to kill arises from their role. It provides intimate contact with vulnerable clients and a trusted position in the community. Workers have access to drugs and possess knowledge of how they work. They understand how medical services operate and know the routines of medical facilities.

An assassin may take advantage of the victim's routines and preferences to create the opportunity for carrying out the killing.

Terrorist attacks against members of the public seize the opportunity of comparatively free access to stores, public places with little supervision, and busy transport networks.

Perpetrators using chemical weapons can create opportunities and improve their chance of success. Military personnel can minimise the risk to themselves by initiating an early morning raid, attacking under cover of darkness, and using rockets (rather than manned aircraft) to deliver chemical agents. Pre-bombardment can create opportunities for inflicting maximum damage by driving people underground before attacking them with heavier-than-air poison gases.

For mass suicides in cults, opportunity arises when members are isolated from the rest of society. This can be achieved by keeping cult members on the move, maintaining anonymity, using fake identities, and by occupying a private, secluded, or remote site. Such steps enable leaders to exert pressure on members to comply with the demands of the cult.

Capital punishment gives a different emphasis to the understanding of opportunity. An executioner does not (like a criminal perpetrator) plan and create a personal opportunity to kill. The date and time are set in advance by a legal process, and the execution is carried out according to protocols.

Location

Predictably, the location of healthcare serial poisoning is the medical facility at which the worker is employed. Where a perpetrator frequently changes their place of work, this can conceal wrongdoing. A physician may use a home visit to commit murder when the patient is alone and unsupervised by others.

With assassination, location is likely chosen to allow the poisoning to be carried out unnoticed or little noticed and to enable the perpetrator to escape.

Terrorist attacks using poison tend to favour accessible and regularly used locations (stores, transport systems) which allow perpetrators to introduce poison, ensuring that the public are affected soon after.

In warfare locations, for deploying chemical weapons are chosen strategically. They may be an enemy stronghold, a highly contested area, or an enemy weapons supply route.

Location in cult mass suicides tends to be separated from others who might subvert the cult message or mission. This might be a private gated community or a remote isolated site.

With capital punishment, normally, the location is a prison. Within it, usually near the condemned cell, is a dedicated space that meets protocol requirements for execution by gas chamber or lethal injection. In its design, the execution chamber may enable relatives and others to witness the procedure and allow the prisoner to make a final statement.

Perpetrator–Victim Relationship

In healthcare serial poisoning, the perpetrator–victim relationship of health practitioner and patient both allows access to potential victims and protects the perpetrator from suspicion. Victims are often ill (but may be recovering) and may be elderly. Perpetrators tend not to select victims according to any social, occupational, or ethnic pattern.

With political assassinations, victim and perpetrator characteristics may be similar if they have military or intelligence backgrounds. Usually there is no direct personal relationship between perpetrator and victim, but where there is, it can be used to the assassin's advantage.

Terrorists usually have no personal connection to victims. Terrorists identify groups for ideological reasons, or people simply going about their daily business. In organised terrorist groups, members may be highly educated and deployed according to their specialist knowledge and skills.

In wartime, enemies may dispute territory, revenge a previous attack on their own forces, or carry out 'ethnic cleansing' (usually related to territory). Victims can be men, women, and children, civilians, or military personnel. Groups may be defined ethnically or according to whether they are considered a threat.

Cult leaders are perpetrators in guiding or driving members to mass suicide. Their demographic details—age, sex, ethnicity, social, and educational background—may be less influential than other factors. Leaders may be charismatic and persuasive. But they may experience mental disorder, hold irrational views, and demonstrate a thirst for power. Cult members can be both victims of the leader's beliefs and perpetrators of their own deaths. Their demographics may reflect the group's aims and values. Where sex is forbidden, child members are unlikely. A cult espousing racial equality may attract a high proportion of minority ethnic members. Where a group lives together, sustaining itself for long periods, members will likely have a variety of skills and occupations. A common thread, relating to recruitment, is members' interest in the spiritual or esoteric and belief in a possible afterlife.

No personal perpetrator–victim relationship exists with capital punishment. In criminal homicide, there are different perpetrator–victim demographic patterns, for example with male on male general homicides or femicide (Brookman 2005, pp. 122, 141). These are absent in executions because it involves a legal, not a personal, connection. Prisoner demographics may reflect social inequities, so a higher-than-expected proportion of poor people or members of ethnic minorities may face execution. Also, many countries preclude a child being culpable of crime and liable for execution. However, the executioner does not select those to be killed on any such criteria but acts according to a legal duty.

Overall, means, motive, opportunity, location, and perpetrator–victim relationship are influenced by the context and may be actively chosen by the perpetrator to suit the context.

Evasion and Response in Different Contexts

Healthcare Serial Poisoning

Evasion

A healthcare serial poisoner's workplace may be relatively isolated from public gaze in a care home, nursing home, hospital ward, physician's surgery, clinic, or patient's own home. They have legitimate access to facilities, medication, and patients. Perpetrators can avoid suspicion by murdering through interfering with a patient's correct drug dose to mimic signs and symptoms of the patient's illness.

To evade scrutiny, a perpetrator sometimes becomes a sole practitioner or moves from job to job. Healthcare serial poisoners can use their knowledge of the routines of their workplaces, such as busy or less supervised times, to harm patients with less risk of detection. Perpetrators may falsify their credentials and/or fabricate critical events (Yorker et al. 2006). Someone who gets excitement from 'rescuing' patients, whom they have poisoned, may appear concerned and efficient because they are often available to 'help'. After committing murder, a physician may alter patient (computer) records perhaps by indicating that the patient was ill for weeks or months prior to the killing.

Employers may have weak recruitment procedures or might provide a satisfactory or even a good reference for a worker who has attracted suspicion. When staff express concerns about another worker, employers may not always listen or investigate thoroughly enough. Formal surveillance may be too weak for employers to detect and act on potential early warnings. Even where police enquiries are initiated, investigators may lack the necessary knowledge and expertise to recognise and evaluate the risk.

Response

Several implications arise from how healthcare serial poisoners can avoid detection. Employment recruitment procedures need to be rigorous and comprehensive and the reasons for a would-be employer's frequent changes of job should be examined carefully. References from one employer to another potential employer should be honest about any concerns. (Some US states have adopted laws giving immunity to employers providing truthful and frank appraisals.) Procedures for staff raising concerns about another employer need to be strong and supported by an open (but not overly suspicious) culture. Formal oversight and supervision of employees should be serious and thorough. Where investigations are initiated by employers, those undertaking them whether internally or externally must have the necessary expertise and support. Healthcare employers should consider fraud or misrepresentation as a serious risk factor in patient safety.

Ramsland (2007) examined perpetrators' characteristics, motives, and methods and developed a checklist of features associated with healthcare serial killing. These included 'Moves from one hospital to another', 'Prefers night shifts—fewer colleagues about', 'Predicts when someone will die', and 'Appears to have a personality disorder'. Some items were found to particularly common in cases of nurses convicted of serially killing patients (Yardley and Wilson 2016), and included 'Higher incidences of death on his/her shift', 'History of mental instability/depression', and 'Makes colleagues anxious/suspicious'. Such checklists can raise awareness of behaviours and traits among healthcare workers that might compromise patient safety. However, the brevity of some items can be misleading.

Assassination

Evasion

Assassins are trained and may be supported by a network of others helping with planning, travel arrangements, weapons, escape routes, and documentation such as false passports.

Planning includes enabling the assassin to gain access to the target or their close surroundings and escaping usually in a prearranged route. Suspicion and surveillance are side-stepped when poison is used unobtrusively. It might be discretely added to the victim's drink in a hotel or delivered by a concealed weapon. Natural surveillance is ineffective because no one is aware of a notable incident. Dupes unsuspected by the target may be blackmailed, persuaded, or tricked into carrying out an assassination by puppet masters. This can enable an assassination to be performed in plain sight in a public place. An attack might take place in an airport where a victim's personal security might be relaxed because of the existing perimeter of airport security. With poisoning on foreign soil, domestic restrictions on their possession are circumvented by assassins smuggling poisons and associated weapons into the country, or by their using binary chemicals.

Victims themselves and authorities who might offer them protection may not know that a target of assassination is at risk. Where someone is a known risk, they may employ private security staff or be guarded by authorities but ineffectively. Authorities may be unaware of preparations for an assassination, even of recent previous attempts because of insufficient oversight of the target or failures in intelligence gathering. Signs of heightened risk may be missed such as a potential victim increasing public criticism of an oppressive hostile regime.

Response

Preventing an assassination firstly requires that the target and authorities are aware of the risk of a possible attack and of any imminent attack. This also applies to any personal security detail employed by the target. Knowledge of a possible attack may come through state intelligence or private sources. Also, it may be inferred by authorities that the subject's actions such as criticising a hostile regime are increasing the likelihood of attack. Security arrangements may then be enhanced. The target may themselves move, or authorities may move them to a secret location.

If a target survives an assassination attempt, authorities have a second opportunity to protect them and may arrange transfer to a safe house and increase their protection. Where a primary subject has been attacked, authorities can still take precautionary actions with potential secondary targets. Police and the media can warn the public to be especially alert. Members of the public may be advised to avoid certain at-risk areas, for example those which might be contaminated with poison. Even further removed from existing assassinations are attempts to discourage future attacks including copycat ones. Authorities seek to do this by revealing some details of the modus operandi and identifying the perpetrators. Politicians may also retaliate against the country suspected of being behind the attack, usually by diplomatic expulsions or economic sanctions.

Terrorism

Evasion

Terrorists seek success in their terms, by choosing targets that are exposed, vital, iconic, legitimate, destructible, occupied, nearer, and easy. Terrorists choose weapons that are multipurpose, undetectable, removable, destructive, enjoyable, reliable, obtainable, uncomplicated, and safe. They use tools such as secretly produced poison. Terrorists will seek facilitating conditions making attacks easy, safe, excusable, enticing, and rewarding (Clarke and Newman 2006).

Using the easy public access to stores, terrorists poison or threaten to poison consumables like loose groceries where detection is difficult. They attack places having open public access such as transport systems. They can deposit poison and get away because targets, unaware of any attack, neither escape nor notice the attacker. Terrorists may use homemade poisons or factory manufactured ones if they are part of a large organisation. Transport, planning, and other arrangements are made by terrorist organisations to facilitate the attack and avoid detection. In terrorist organisations, secrecy, high internal security, and encrypted communications can conceal plots from authorities. Such secrecy also allows the organisation to indoctrinate members. Internet sites encouraging terrorism and recruiting individuals may be on the dark web and hidden by other means. Because terrorist targets may be random members of the public, it is difficult for authorities to know who will be targeted as there is no personal direct motive.

Response

Recall the likely efforts of terrorists to ensure success in their terms, by preferences for certain targets, weapons, tools, and facilitating conditions (Clarke and Newman 2006). Implications for prevention include recognising and better protecting higher-risk targets such as certain groups (e.g. ethnic, religious, and homosexual) and vulnerable venues (e.g. night clubs, places of worship, and schools). Also important is using any specific intelligence and being aware of continuing risks (e.g. plots involving adaptations of product tampering).

Authorities were unable to stop early examples of product tampering but developed packaging which helped to prevent further attacks. Police and the media warned about the risk of copycat crimes to alert members of the public and storekeepers. Also, US legislation made product tampering a serious offense attracting heavy punishment. On transport systems, authorities are now better at screening entrances and exits. Security services and police use intelligence information to try to stop attacks by monitoring a suspect's communications (including the internet and telephone) or by detaining suspects. Police investigating attacks may be able to find a pattern and prevent further deaths. Authorities monitor internet sites to identify corrosive propaganda and investigate its sources.

Authorities must find a balance between, on the one hand, concealing information that might assist further terrorism and, on the other hand, informing the public and revealing aspects of the modus operandi to discourage further attacks.

Warfare

Evasion

Countries may falsely claim to have no chemical weapons. If it is known that a country has or had such weapons, it may agree to destroy them and then not comply, or falsely state that it has already destroyed them. A country may deny using chemical weapons and accuse opponents including other countries of fabricating accounts to justify some hostile action of their own.

When chemical weapons are used in warfare, perpetrators ignore international agreements banning their manufacture and use. While this happens with international conflicts, it is easier when there is a civil war and 'outside' countries are not directly involved. The country and its allies can deny their involvement and sometimes can convincingly place the blame on opposition forces. Where state actors are involved, they can evade controls by using wealth or political positioning to manufacture or otherwise acquire chemical weapons.

Errant countries also seek to evade inspections of facilities and sites of suspected attacks. Countries can deny access to international inspectors or delay their access to allow time to clean up an area. They can allow access to inspectors from ally countries who may give a more favourable account. Where inspections following a suspected attack find environmental samples of chemicals, the country can attempt to explain this by claiming that the chemicals came from a legitimate chemical factory that was accidentally damaged.

Response

From 1997, a Chemical Weapons Convention prohibited developing, producing, stockpiling, transferring, and using chemical weapons and their precursors. Relatedly, the Organisation for the Prohibition of Chemical Weapons verifies the destruction of chemical weapons. In warfare affected or concerned parties may cite such conventions and provide evidence of non-compliance. In conflicts, including ones where chemical weapons may be used, international bodies try to settle disputes or at least de-escalate tensions. Safety zones may be agreed where civilians can shelter to avoid being targeted.

Potential targets of chemical weapons, whether troops or civilians, may wear protective clothing and equipment. Gas masks with chemical filters are effective against inhaled chemical agents and protect the eyes. Wearing a protective garment guards against chemical weapons that harm the skin upon contact (Shea 2013, p. 8). Targeted individuals and groups may shelter in specially deployed buildings. They may receive training about what to do if there is a chemical attack including where to go and how to use equipment. All this requires planning and resources.

After the event, evidence of chemical attacks may be gathered from various sources. These include eyewitness reports, personal phone camera recordings put on social media platforms, satellite images, post-mortem examinations of victims, environmental samples, and thorough site inspections. Such information aims to publicise what has happened, bring perpetrators to justice, and deter others from using chemical weapons. Other states may make deterrent retaliatory attacks using conventional weapons against a state or regime that has used chemical weapons.

Mass Suicide Cults

Evasion

Cult leaders may avoid scrutiny by aiming their message directly at those likely to respond, through groups already interested in spiritual and esoteric matters, and by having recruitment meetings in private homes. A cult may target vulnerable or gullible people. They may avoid reporters who could present the cult negatively and leaders may even go into hiding. Where a cult has gradually become corrupted, leaders may trade off its initial respectability.

Leaders may try to isolate the group from the influences of wider society through keeping people on the move, or by staying in private, or inaccessible places. They may ensure that members do not question the cult's message through exerting different types of influence. Examples are group teaching, peer pressure to conform, developing strict routines and rules, encouraging confession where rules have been broken, and expelling dissenters. Other strategies include encouraging secrecy and security consciousness and representing the outside world and wider society to members as threatening or dangerous to the cult's cause. Leaders may introduce 'controlling' rules encouraging members to be incurious and self-effacing and to distrust their own judgement. Allocated partners may watch over each other's obedience. Access to money and its use may be strictly controlled. Clothing may be shared. Sex may be forbidden. Where cult members travel outside the cult compound, it may be under strict rules and involve secret communications with the leaders. If members work in the wider community, they may use fictionalised job applications, false resumes, and fake references.

Response

Pre-emptively, authorities and representatives of the media may draw attention to the negative aspects of cults. This may involve encouraging public scrutiny, airing negative publicity, and challenging the cult's message. Authorities may draw these aspects to the attention of individuals who might be vulnerable to a cult's attractions. Leaders of the main world faiths may warn of the risks associated with cults. Authorities can try to make possible recruits aware of harmful features such as injunctions and rules aimed at discouraging members' critical or independent thinking.

Relatives and friends occasionally forcibly abduct potential cult recruits. Members who have themselves escaped a cult may temporarily stay in a refuge or private place. Authorities may monitor the communications of cults including their websites or advertisements aiming to recruit new members. Relatives, friends, and others may alert authorities about concerns. They may press for cult's actions to be investigated or their premises to be inspected. Concerned parties may contact the police, hire detectives, and encourage journalists to investigate. Where a cult member becomes a whistle-blower (including via relatives), any claims should be properly investigated. At the same time, authorities need to be aware that investigations can precipitate dangerous responses from cult leaders such as fleeing to a remote area or a different country posing an even greater risk to members.

Capital Punishment

Evasion

'Evasion' here refers to efforts to avoid an offender receiving the death penalty. Opponents of capital punishment may present a range of arguments against it, for example moral, practical, and religious ones.

Lawyers may delay the execution by repeatedly appealing in the expectation that one appeal will succeed, or that new exonerating evidence will emerge. Reasons for appeal are numerous. Using the gas chamber or lethal injection (in the United States) may be unconstitutional. A prisoner's illnesses and possible failed veins could make lethal injection impracticable and lead to a botched or aborted execution. An incapacitating injury after a punishment hearing might reduce a prisoner's ability to cause harm. The prisoner may want to donate non-vital organs. A prisoner's brutal childhood experiences call for clemency. Brain damage may have affected a prisoner's judgement when he killed victims.

Attempts are made to disrupt the supply of gas chamber chemicals and lethal injection drugs. Opponents to capital punishment draw wider public attention to death penalty procedures, citing witnesses and those directly involved in preparing and executing the condemned person. Publicising humanising details, or botched procedures, it is believed might diminish the public appetite for the death penalty. Opponents might publicise the identity of those involved in the execution (including suppliers and manufacturers of the necessary drugs and chemicals) to try to discourage them by exposing them to possible public pressure.

Response

Supporters of capital punishment present it as state-sanctioned legal killing. In the United States, appeals have been declined where they have: questioned the constitutionality of the gas chamber or lethal injection; proposed that a prisoner's condition could make lethal injection impracticable; raised a prisoner's brutal childhood experiences; and claimed that brain damage affected a prisoner's judgement.

Supporters of the death penalty may draw public attention to the heinous nature of the crimes for which the condemned person has been convicted, for example the rape and murder of a child. Sources might be the bereaved relatives, friends, and neighbours. By publicising such information, supporters of the death penalty may believe that public will be shocked by the brutality of the crime and that the public will recognise that capital punishment is justified.

The death penalty ensures that the executed person can never offend again (although counterarguments cite the risk of executing innocent people that cannot then be rectified). Where evidence is unequivocal and the prisoner convincingly admits the crime, arguments that the wrong person is to be executed assume less power. Supporters may claim that the death penalty, if carried out without undue delay, is a deterrent to others from committing similar crimes, although opponents claim that there is no deterrent effect or a limited effect. Different ways of presenting evidence are used to support positions. Death penalty proponents may point out that most of the world's population live in jurisdictions supporting the death sentence, so the majority view prevails. Opponents emphasise that most *countries* do not have the death penalty, highlighting that most legislatures oppose it.

References

Brookman, F. (2005). *Understanding Homicide*. London and Los Angeles: Sage.
Clarke, R. V. G., & Newman, G. R. (2006). *Outsmarting the Terrorists*. Westport, CT: ABC-CLIO.
Farrell, M. (2018). *Criminology of Serial Poisoners*. London: Palgrave Macmillan.
Ramsland, K. (2007). *Inside the Minds of Healthcare Serial Killers: Why They Kill*. Westport, CT: Praeger.
Shea, D. A. (2013). *Chemical Weapons: A Summary Report of Characteristics and Effects* Washington, DC, Congressional Research Service 7-5700 (13 September 2013) www.crs.gov RS42862 and https://fas.org/sgp/crs/nuke/R42862.pdf.

Yardley, E., & Wilson, D. (2016). In Search of the 'Angels of Death': Conceptualising the Contemporary Nurse Healthcare Serial Killer. *Journal of Investigative Psychology and Offender Profiling, 13*(1), 39–55.

Yorker, B. C., Kizer, K. W., Lampe, P., Forest, A. R. W., Lannan, J. M., & Russell, D. A. (2006). Serial Murder by Healthcare Professionals. *Journal of Forensic Science, 51*(6), 1–10.

Index

© The Author(s) 2020
M. Farrell, *Criminology of Poisoning Contexts*,
https://doi.org/10.1007/978-3-030-40830-5

CPI Antony Rowe
Eastbourne, UK
March 18, 2020